TWO-STEP | DIABETES COOKBOOK

NANCY S. HUGHES

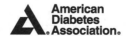

Director, Book Publishing, Abe Ogden; *Managing Editor,* Greg Guthrie; *Acquisitions Editor,* Victor Van Beuren; *Editor,* Rebekah Renshaw; *Production Manager,* Melissa Sprott; *Composition,* Circle Graphics; *Cover Design,* Vis á Vis Creative Concepts; *Photography,* Renee Comet; *Printer,* R.R. Donnelley.

Printed in the United States of America
1 3 5 7 9 10 8 6 4 2

The suggestions and information contained in this publication are generally consistent with the *Standard of Medical Care in Diabetes* and other policies of the American Diabetes Association, but they do not represent the policy or position of the Association or any of its boards or committees. Reasonable steps have been taken to ensure the accuracy of the information presented. However, the American Diabetes Association cannot ensure the safety or efficacy of any product or service described in this publication. Individuals are advised to consult a physician or other appropriate health care professional before undertaking any diet or exercise program or taking any medication referred to in this publication. Professionals must use and apply their own professional judgment, experience, and training and should not rely solely on the information contained in this publication before prescribing any diet, exercise, or medication. The American Diabetes Association—its officers, directors, employees, volunteers, and members—assumes no responsibility or liability for personal or other injury, loss, or damage that may result from the suggestions or information in this publication.

♾ The paper in this publication meets the requirements of the ANSI Standard Z39.48-1992 (permanence of paper).

ADA titles may be purchased for business or promotional use or for special sales. To purchase more than 50 copies of this book at a discount, or for custom editions of this book with your logo, contact the American Diabetes Association at the address below or at booksales@diabetes.org.

American Diabetes Association
1701 North Beauregard Street
Alexandria, Virginia 22311

DOI: 10.2337/9781580405621

Library of Congress Cataloging-in-Publication Data

Hughes, Nancy S.
  Two-step diabetes cookbook / Nancy S. Hughes.
    pages cm
  Includes bibliographical references and index.
  ISBN 978-1-58040-562-1 (alk. paper)
  1. Diabetes--Diet therapy--Recipes. I. American Diabetes Association. II. Title.
  RC662.H85 2015
  641.5'6314--dc23
                          2015002633

TABLE OF CONTENTS

BREAKFAST

LUNCH

Soups

Salads

Sandwiches

APPETIZERS, SNACKS

SIDE SALADS

SIDES (VEGETABLES AND FRUITS AND GRAINS)

ENTREES

Beef

Pork

Poultry

Seafood

DEDICATION

To my children: Will, Annie, and Taft; their spouses: Kelly, Terry, and Kara; and to my grandchildren: Molly Catherine, Anna Flynn, and Baby Hughes, Jilli, Jesse, and Emma. You're being exposed to new foods, new recipes every single time you walk through my doors. Thank you for your enthusiasm, your honesty...and, well, for just being you...each in your own special way!

To my husband, Greg: You are as much fun to be around now as you were when we first met...you're still hilarious! Thanks for the fun you bring and the calm you give when calm is not part of my vocabulary...stay close!

Love, me

ACKNOWLEDGMENTS

To Will Hughes, my chef, my "on task" guy, and my son. You're an asset to my business that I just didn't imagine could happen…two Hughes's working together cohesively under one roof, with one goal. It's working…and it's working very well!

To Melanie McKibbin, my business manager, you always come with a smile on your face and always know how to "untangle" and make sense out of the mounds of paperwork waiting for you, then you turn around and handle…everything I don't want to do!

To Sylvia Vollmer, my "always-there-for-me" assistant, who I can count on now and always…and I appreciate that more than you realize!

To Abe Ogden, director of book publishing; Victor Van Beuren, acquisitions editor; and Rebekah Renshaw, my editor: how many times can I say thank you for being there for me…listening, laughing, and dining together. I'd say that's a perfect combination all the way around!

PREFACE

I could never understand why my mother always told me to keep things simple when company was coming. I wanted to make extravagant meals, clean closets, and polish…the roof! Why? I'm not sure, actually, I just thought that's what was "expected" when company was coming.

But the reason she told me to keep things simple was because when things are simple, I am calm and when I am calm, I am able to truly enjoy the company that's coming, rather than have silly questions swirling around in my head, like "Did I polish the silver…enough?"

Life is moving quickly and if we don't *hurry up* and s-l-o-w d-o-w-n, we'll miss the best parts…hope you enjoy all your parts…AND these recipes waiting for you!

"I Hope You're Hungry!"

N

A WORD FROM THE AUTHOR

I have zero patience for complicated recipes…my life is confusing enough without added stress!!

Even now…after _years_ of cooking, writing, and teaching, I look at a new recipe with a long list of directions, and I literally feel like I want to take a nap…I am mentally "exhausted." Don't misunderstand, there's a time and place for lengthy, multiple-step recipes—on the weekends possibly, but on a regular day, I want simple, I want comfort, AND I want it to be delicious!

So in order to achieve that "simple" mealtime style, I've created 150 recipes for busy, health-conscious people with or _without_ diabetes who want recipes that have straightforward, easy-to-follow directions…2-STEP directions, to be precise! Every single recipe follows the guidelines of the American Diabetes Association while providing tons of flavor and comfort!

As with all my books with the American Diabetes Association, the recipes are mainstream and family-friendly, using ingredients that are found in your local grocery stores. In other words, "normal" ingredients!

In just a matter of minutes, your meals will be on the table in a flash with energy left over to actually enjoy those meals…and relax!

One thing I discovered while creating these recipes was the importance of...

RETHINKING

When planning out your own recipes and menus, always ask yourself: "Now, how can I make this simpler? Can I pull something out of the freezer, open a can from the pantry, or rip open a package of lettuce and other veggies?"

Certain items that can actually save you money and a world of time and energy while keeping you on the right path, are items like:

- Rotisserie chickens (buy 2 and keep one in the freezer for backup!)
- Hard-boiled eggs (already cooked and peeled for you).
- Premade healthy yogurt-based dips for veggies (great for wraps, too).
- Sliced-to-order deli items, such as roast beef, lean ham, or a specific cheese, saving you from having to buy more than you will actually use for a particular recipe.

Walk The Aisles:
Don't overlook the canned, packaged, and frozen aisles...you don't have to always rely on fresh. Frozen and canned (especially when an ingredient is out of season) can be a great source because they are canned and frozen during their PEAK season...so the nutrients are high and the flavors preserved. There's even frozen and packaged cooked brown rice and sweet potato fries on the shelves waiting for you right now!

Find Multitaskers:
Use multitasking ingredients. These are "everyday" ingredients that you can make work for you in more ways than the traditional way...stir some in and spoon a small amount on top at the end for a more pronounced flavor. Just be careful of the sodium

and fat when using the following (just a small amount is all you will need to provide a pop of flavor!):

- Picante sauce and salsa
- Pizza sauce
- Turkey pepperoni
- Turkey or chicken sausage
- Olives, pepperoncini, banana peppers
- High-flavored cheeses, such as reduced-fat feta, blue cheese, sharp cheddar, or pepper jack
- Pesto, such as basil or sun-dried tomato

Split It Up:

There are tons of dried herbs, spices, and salt-free seasoning blends on the shelves, but it can become rather costly when you think you'll only be in need of a small amount. That's when you go in with a friend or family member who might want to split the container...it's like buying the seasoning for half the price!

THE IMPORTANCE OF STOCKING UP AND HOW

If you can do one thing…this is what I _highly_ suggest: "Keep it stocked". PERIOD.

Keep items on hand (in your freezer, fridge, and pantry) that you can always fall back on for 3–4 breakfasts, lunches, dinners…and don't forget snacks! That way, it will keep you on a healthy track while keeping your food budget on track, too!

It's so easy to "drive through" or "order in," but the calories, fat grams, carbs, _and_ the cost factor all add up FAST!! Keep ingredients for those "fast food favorites" on hand, such as burgers, fries, pizza, and tacos. Then you'll look forward to actually making them because you have all the ingredients right there…stocked! There's absolutely **no** excuse to look elsewhere…it's ready, it's waiting, and it's healthier, too!

SHORTCUTTING IN THE KITCHEN

- **CITRUS JUICE:** When you're juicing lemons or limes, juice more than the recipe calls for. Save steps and freeze the extra juice in small snack baggies (lie flat) so you can easily and effortlessly break off what you need rather than thawing the whole bag.

- **CHOPPING ONIONS:** Look over your recipes and menus for the week and chop for all of them, seal it up, and toss in the fridge. You can store it up to 1 week. *Side Tip on Chopping Onions: When chopping onions and you begin to tear, immediately run your knife and your hands under water and you'll stop immediately!*

- **PULL FIRST:** Pull all ingredients for the recipe before you begin preparing that recipe.

- **BEFORE YOU BEGIN:** Prepare the ingredients as listed in the ingredient list, such as chopped, rinsed, and drained, etc., first before you start the directions section of a recipe.

- **PREP AHEAD:** A great time and energy saver is to prep 3–4 dinner recipes at one time, store them in the fridge until needed, then all you have to do is take 2-steps and eat!

- **SALAD SENSE:** Why mess up two dishes when making a salad? Often all you need to do is place the salad ingredients in a bowl, sprinkle the ingredients for the salad dressing over the salad, and simply toss together until well blended. One dish, no extra washing OR steps! It's simple, make it easy on yourself!

- **SKILLET SERVE:** Use your skillet as the serving piece. It keeps the food hotter than transferring it to a serving platter and cuts down on cleanup and time spent (it is a great step-saver and one less dish to wash!).

- **COOKING IN STAGES:** When adding raw veggies (or shrimp) to pasta, rice, or other grain dishes, save steps by adding them to the pot 3–4 minutes before the pasta, rice, or other grain is done. They cook together, which means 1 pot to wash and you can drain all at once...steps saved!

JUST ONE MORE THING . . .

Keep this thought in the back of your mind when preparing your own creations:

"The more you can put in a bowl at one time, the easier it will _feel_ to make that dish!"

In other words, "COMBINE ALL" whenever possible. It saves on dishes to clean, then you'll want to go back to that recipe again and again! And THAT'S what keeps you on track!!

I Hope You're Hungry!

—N

BREAKFAST

Mexican Skillet Egg Casserole

1 teaspoon canola oil

1 1/2 cups egg substitute

1 (4.5-ounce) can chopped green chilies, drained

1/3 cup shredded reduced-fat sharp cheddar cheese

1 (2.25-ounce) can sliced ripe olives, drained

1/2 cup diced tomatoes

1 ripe medium avocado, peeled, pitted, and chopped

1/4 cup chopped fresh cilantro

1 Heat the oil in a medium nonstick skillet over medium heat. Add the eggs, cook 1 minute, and gently stir until just set (Note: eggs will still be very wet). Remove from heat.

2 Top with the remaining ingredient in the order given. Cover and cook over medium-low heat 2–3 minutes or until cheese melts.

EXCHANGES / CHOICES

1/2 Carbohydrate
2 Protein, lean
1 Fat

BASIC NUTRITIONAL VALUES

Calories	160	**Potassium**	410 mg
Calories from Fat	80	**Total Carbohydrate**	9 g
Total Fat	9.0 g	Dietary Fiber	4 g
Saturated Fat	2.0 g	Sugars	2 g
Trans Fat	0.0 g	**Protein**	13 g
Cholesterol	5 mg	**Phosphorus**	90 mg
Sodium	355 mg		

Breakfast Cookies

Serves: 12
Serving Size: 1 cookie

1 1/3 **cups** quick-cooking oats
1/2 **cup** white whole-wheat flour
1/4 **cup** ground flax meal
1 **cup** slivered almonds
1 **cup** reduced-sugar dried cranberries
1 **teaspoon** cinnamon
1/2 **teaspoon** salt
1/2 **cup** egg substitute
1/3 **cup** packed brown sugar substitute blend, such as Splenda
1/4 **cup** canola oil
1 **teaspoon** almond extract

1. Preheat oven to 350°F. Meanwhile, stir together all ingredients in a large bowl. Spoon mixture to make 12 mounds on a large nonstick baking sheet coated with cooking spray.

2. Bake 13 minutes or until beginning to lightly brown on edges. Place baking sheet on wire rack and cool 2 minutes before removing. Cool completely.

Cook's Tip: Serve each cookie with 1/2 cup nonfat plain Greek yogurt for a high fiber, protein-filled "on the go" breakfast!

EXCHANGES / CHOICES
2 Carbohydrate
2 Fat

BASIC NUTRITIONAL VALUES

Calories	215	**Potassium**	160 mg
Calories from Fat	100	**Total Carbohydrate**	28 g
Total Fat	11.0 g	Dietary Fiber	6 g
Saturated Fat	0.9 g	Sugars	8 g
Trans Fat	0.0 g	**Protein**	5 g
Cholesterol	0 mg	**Phosphorus**	110 mg
Sodium	120 mg		

Sausage, Sage, and Hash Brown Casserole

SERVES: 6
SERVING SIZE: 1⅓ cups

4 ounces reduced-fat breakfast sausage
1½ cups diced yellow onions
1½ pounds frozen hash brown potatoes
1 cup reduced-fat 98% fat-free cream of chicken soup
1 cup fat-free Greek yogurt
1 tablespoon canola oil
¼ cup chopped fresh parsley
½ to 1 teaspoon dried sage
¼ teaspoon black pepper
1½ ounces shredded reduced-fat sharp cheddar cheese
¼ teaspoon salt

1 Preheat oven to 350°F. Heat a large nonstick skillet over medium heat until hot. Add the sausage and cook 2 minutes, breaking up larger pieces while cooking. Stir in the onions and cook 3 minutes or until onions are beginning to brown and are tender-crisp. Remove from heat.

2 Stir in potatoes, soup, yogurt, oil, parsley, sage, and black pepper. Cover and bake 1 hour or until potatoes are tender. Sprinkle with cheese and salt. Cover and let stand 10 minutes to develop flavors.

EXCHANGES / CHOICES
1½ Starch
1 Vegetable
1 Protein, lean
1 Fat

BASIC NUTRITIONAL VALUES

Calories	235	**Potassium**	590 mg
Calories from Fat	70	**Total Carbohydrate**	31 g
Total Fat	8.0 g	Dietary Fiber	4 g
Saturated Fat	2.4 g	Sugars	4 g
Trans Fat	0.0 g	**Protein**	12 g
Cholesterol	15 mg	**Phosphorus**	190 mg
Sodium	545 mg		

Pumpkin Pie Oatmeal

SERVES: 4
SERVING SIZE: $^2/_3$ cup

1 Heat a small skillet over medium-high heat, add nuts and cook 2 minutes or until beginning to lightly brown, stirring frequently.

2 Place nuts in a medium microwave-safe bowl with remaining ingredient. Cover and microwave on high for 2 minutes. Stir and microwave for another 2 minutes or until heated.

2 ounces chopped pecans, toasted
1 $^1/_4$ cups quick-cooking rolled oats
1 $^1/_4$ cups fat-free milk
$^3/_4$ cup canned pumpkin puree
1 teaspoon ground cinnamon
$^1/_4$ teaspoon ground nutmeg
2 tablespoons sugar
$^1/_8$ teaspoon salt
1 teaspoon vanilla, butter, and nut flavoring, or **1 $^1/_2$ teaspoons** vanilla

EXCHANGES / CHOICES	BASIC NUTRITIONAL VALUES			
1 $^1/_2$ Starch	**Calories**	270	**Potassium**	370 mg
$^1/_2$ Milk, fat-free	Calories from Fat	110	**Total Carbohydrate**	34 g
$^1/_2$ Carbohydrate	**Total Fat**	12.0 g	Dietary Fiber	6 g
1 $^1/_2$ Fat	Saturated Fat	1.3 g	Sugars	13 g
	Trans Fat	0.0 g	**Protein**	8 g
	Cholesterol	0 mg	**Phosphorus**	240 mg
	Sodium	110 mg		

Day or Night Italian Scramble

1 **cup** grape tomatoes, quartered
16 pitted kalamata olives, coarsely chopped
$^1/_4$ **cup** chopped fresh basil or arugula
1 **tablespoon** extra virgin olive oil, divided use
1 **teaspoon** cider vinegar
2 **cups** egg substitute
1 **ounce** crumbled reduced-fat feta cheese

1 Combine the tomatoes, olives, basil, 2 teaspoons oil, and vinegar in a small bowl and set aside.

2 Heat the remaining 1 teaspoon oil in a medium nonstick skillet over medium heat, tilting to coat lightly. Add the egg substitute and cook 1 minute without stirring. Then gently stir eggs until just set. Remove from heat and top with the tomato mixture and feta.

EXCHANGES / CHOICES

$^1/_2$ Carbohydrate
2 Protein, lean
$^1/_2$ Fat

BASIC NUTRITIONAL VALUES

Calories	140	**Potassium**	300 mg
Calories from Fat	65	**Total Carbohydrate**	5 g
Total Fat	7.0 g	Dietary Fiber	1 g
Saturated Fat	1.3 g	Sugars	2 g
Trans Fat	0.0 g	**Protein**	14 g
Cholesterol	5 mg	**Phosphorus**	55 mg
Sodium	440 mg		

Handheld Apple Breakfast Rounds

SERVES: 8
SERVING SIZE: 1 round

1 Stir together the peanut butter, cream cheese, and honey in a small bowl until well blended. Spoon 1 tablespoon of the mixture evenly over each apple round. Sprinkle evenly with the cereal and nuts.

$^1/_3$ **cup** reduced-fat peanut butter
3 tablespoons fat-free cream cheese
1 tablespoon honey
2 medium Granny Smith apples
   (12 ounces), cored and sliced
   crosswise into 8 rounds total
$^1/_2$ **cup** high-fiber shredded cereal
$^1/_4$ **cup** slivered almonds, preferably
   toasted

COOK'S TIP: Double the recipe to keep on hand in refrigerator for a "hurry-up-and-go" breakfast!

EXCHANGES / CHOICES
1 Carbohydrate
1 Fat

BASIC NUTRITIONAL VALUES

Calories	125	**Potassium**	180 mg
Calories from Fat	55	**Total Carbohydrate**	17 g
Total Fat	6.0 g	Dietary Fiber	4 g
Saturated Fat	0.8 g	Sugars	8 g
Trans Fat	0.0 g	**Protein**	4 g
Cholesterol	0 mg	**Phosphorus**	105 mg
Sodium	120 mg		

Sausage and Fresh Basil Fast Frittata

SERVES: 4
SERVING SIZE: 1/4 frittata wedge per serving

2 teaspoons extra virgin olive oil

8 ounces chicken with sun-dried tomatoes sausage, diced

1 1/2 cups egg substitute

1 ounce shredded part-skim mozzarella cheese

1/2 cup finely chopped green onion

1 cup diced tomatoes

1/4 cup chopped fresh basil or flat leaf parsley

1 Heat the oil in a large nonstick skillet over medium heat. Add the sausage and cook 3 minutes or until beginning to brown, stirring occasionally. Pour the egg substitute evenly over the sausage and cook 1 minute. Do not stir. Then, gently lift to allow uncooked egg to flow under. Remove from heat.

2 Sprinkle the cheese, green onions, tomatoes, and basil evenly over all.

EXCHANGES/ CHOICES

1/2 Carbohydrate
3 Protein, lean
1/2 Fat

BASIC NUTRITIONAL VALUES

Calories	190	**Potassium**	425 mg
Calories from Fat	70	**Total Carbohydrate**	6 g
Total Fat	8.0 g	Dietary Fiber	1 g
Saturated Fat	24 g	Sugars	4 g
Trans Fat	0.0 g	**Protein**	21 g
Cholesterol	50 mg	**Phosphorus**	170 mg
Sodium	525 mg		

Ham and Red Pepper Cheddar'd Grits

1 Heat the oil in a medium nonstick skillet over medium-high heat. Tilt skillet to coat bottom lightly and brown the ham, stirring occasionally. Add the peppers and onions and cook 2 minutes or until peppers are tender-crisp. Stir in the margarine. Set aside in a medium bowl and cover to keep warm.

2 Bring the water to a boil in the skillet over medium-high heat. Stir in the grits, garlic powder, and salt. Cook according to package directions. Remove from heat, sprinkle evenly with the cheese, and top with the ham mixture. Do not stir.

$^1/_2$ **teaspoon** canola oil
4 ounces extra-lean diced ham
1 cup finely chopped red bell pepper
$^1/_2$ **cup** finely chopped green onion
1 teaspoon lower-fat (50% vegetable oil) margarine
2 $^1/_2$ cups water
$^1/_2$ **cup** quick-cooking grits
$^1/_4$ **teaspoon** garlic powder
$^1/_8$ **teaspoon** salt
2 ounces reduced-fat shredded sharp cheddar cheese

EXCHANGES / CHOICES	BASIC NUTRITIONAL VALUES			
1 Starch	**Calories**	175	**Potassium**	235 mg
1 Vegetable	Calories from Fat	55	**Total Carbohydrate**	20 g
1 Protein, lean	**Total Fat**	6.0 g	Dietary Fiber	1 g
$^1/_2$ Fat	Saturated Fat	24 g	Sugars	2 g
	Trans Fat	0.0 g	**Protein**	12 g
	Cholesterol	25 mg	**Phosphorus**	165 mg
	Sodium	545 mg		

Apple-Walnut French Toast

6 ounces multi-grain Italian bread, cut in 4 slices

1 cup egg substitute

2 tablespoons plus **2 teaspoons** pure maple syrup

1 cup diced apples

2 ounces chopped walnuts

1 Preheat oven to 450°F. Meanwhile, place the bread in a 13 × 9-inch baking pan, pour the egg substitute over all, and turn several times until the bread slices are completely coated and egg mixture is used. (Let stand in baking pan while oven is preheating.) Place bread slices on baking sheet coated with cooking spray.

2 Bake 6 minutes, turn, and bake 5 minutes or until golden on the bottom. Serve topped with equal amounts of the syrup, apples, and nuts.

COOK'S TIP: Drizzle the syrup on top of the toast before topping with the apples and nuts for peak flavors and sweetness.

EXCHANGES / CHOICES

1 1/2 Starch
1 Carbohydrate
1 Protein, lean
1 1/2 Fat

BASIC NUTRITIONAL VALUES

Calories	285	**Potassium**	300 mg
Calories from Fat	100	**Total Carbohydrate**	34 g
Total Fat	11.0 g	Dietary Fiber	5 g
Saturated Fat	1.3 g	Sugars	15 g
Trans Fat	0.0 g	**Protein**	14 g
Cholesterol	0 mg	**Phosphorus**	160 mg
Sodium	295 mg		

SERVES: 4

SERVING SIZE: 1 shortcake, $1/2$ cup berry mixture, and about 2 tablespoons yogurt per serving

1 Preheat oven to 425°F. Meanwhile, combine the fruit, 1 tablespoon of the sugar substitute, and $1/2$ teaspoon almond extract and set aside.

2 Combine the baking mix, $1/3$ cup of the yogurt, oil, remaining sugar substitute, and extract in a medium bowl. Spoon onto a nonstick baking sheet coated with cooking spray in 4 mounds. Bake 8 minutes or until golden on bottom. Serve topped with fruit mixture and remaining yogurt.

2 cups fresh or frozen blueberries, thawed

3 tablespoons sugar substitute, divided use

1 teaspoon almond extract, divided use

3/4 cup healthy pancake and baking mix, such as Bisquick Heart Smart

1 cup plain nonfat Greek yogurt, divided use

1 tablespoon canola oil

EXCHANGES / CHOICES

2 Carbohydrate
1 Fat

BASIC NUTRITIONAL VALUES

Calories	190	**Potassium**	135 mg
Calories from Fat	45	**Total Carbohydrate**	30 g
Total Fat	5.0 g	Dietary Fiber	2 g
Saturated Fat	0.5 g	Sugars	13 g
Trans Fat	0.0 g	**Protein**	7 g
Cholesterol	5 mg	**Phosphorus**	195 mg
Sodium	260 mg		

Breakfast BLT & E

4 (6-inch) wheat flour tortillas
Nonstick cooking spray
1 cup egg substitute
1/4 **cup** light mayonnaise
4 romaine lettuce leaves, trimmed
6 slices cooked bacon
1 medium tomato, diced
1/4 **cup** chopped fresh cilantro or green
   onion
1 medium lime, quartered

1 Cover tortillas with damp paper towels and set aside.
Coat a 2-cup microwave-safe cup, (such as a Pyrex glass
measuring cup) with cooking spray. Add the egg substitute
and cover and cook 2 minutes. Stir. Place the tortillas
in the microwave alongside the eggs and cook 1 minute
longer or until eggs are just set and tortillas are warmed.

2 Spread each tortilla with 1 tablespoon mayonnaise,
top with a lettuce leaf, 1 1/2 pieces of bacon, and equal
amounts of the egg, tomato, and cilantro. Squeeze lime
juice over all. Fold over sides and cut in half, if desired.
These can also be served open-faced with knife and fork,
if desired.

Cook's Tip: You may purchase precooked bacon in major supermarkets.

EXCHANGES / CHOICES
1 Starch
1/2 Carbohydrate
1 Protein, lean
1 Fat

BASIC NUTRITIONAL VALUES

Calories	210	**Potassium**	315 mg
Calories from Fat	80	**Total Carbohydrate**	21 g
Total Fat	9.0 g	Dietary Fiber	2 g
Saturated Fat	2.2 g	Sugars	3 g
Trans Fat	0.0 g	**Protein**	11 g
Cholesterol	10 mg	**Phosphorus**	90 mg
Sodium	545 mg		

Ham and Swiss Savory French Toast

1 Heat the oil in a large nonstick skillet over medium heat. Meanwhile, dip the bread in the egg substitute, turning to coat until all egg is absorbed.

2 Cook the bread slices 3 minutes. Flip the bread, top each with equal amounts of the mayonnaise, oregano, turkey, green onion, 2 slices tomato, and 3 strips cheese. Cover, reduce heat to medium-low, and cook 3 minutes or until golden on the bottom.

1 tablespoon canola oil

4 ounces multi-grain Italian loaf bread, cut into 4 slices

1 cup egg substitute

2 tablespoons light mayonnaise

1/2 teaspoon dried oregano leaves

2 ounces oven-roasted turkey, chopped, or diced extra-lean ham

1/4 cup finely chopped green onion

8 medium tomato slices

3 very thin slices low-fat Swiss cheese, each cut into 4 strips (12 total strips)

EXCHANGES / CHOICES	BASIC NUTRITIONAL VALUES			
1 Starch	**Calories**	235	**Potassium**	330 mg
2 Protein, lean	Calories from Fat	90	**Total Carbohydrate**	17 g
1 1/2 Fat	**Total Fat**	10.0 g	Dietary Fiber	3 g
	Saturated Fat	2.5 g	Sugars	4 g
	Trans Fat	0.0 g	**Protein**	20 g
	Cholesterol	25 mg	**Phosphorus**	215 mg
	Sodium	330 mg		

Breakfast Egg & Cheese Rounds

4 whole-wheat or multi-grain English muffins, halved

1 **cup** egg substitute

1 **teaspoon** dried oregano leaves

3 **ounces** shredded reduced-fat Italian cheese blend (or **2 ounces** shredded part-skim mozzarella and **2 tablespoons** grated Parmesan cheese)

$^{1}/_{2}$ **cup** diced green bell pepper

$^{1}/_{2}$ **cup** finely chopped red onion

1 Preheat oven to 400°F. Meanwhile, arrange muffins on a baking sheet coated with cooking spray. Spoon 2 tablespoons of the egg over each and top with the remaining ingredients in the order listed.

2 Bake, uncovered, 15 minutes or until eggs are set.

EXCHANGES / CHOICES	BASIC NUTRITIONAL VALUES			
2 Starch	**Calories**	240	**Potassium**	315 mg
2 Protein, lean	Calories from Fat	45	**Total Carbohydrate**	32 g
	Total Fat	5.0 g	Dietary Fiber	5 g
	Saturated Fat	2.5 g	Sugars	7 g
	Trans Fat	0.0 g	**Protein**	18 g
	Cholesterol	10 mg	**Phosphorus**	365 mg
	Sodium	595 mg		

Corn and Potato Breakfast Casserole

1 Preheat oven to 350°F. Meanwhile, combine all ingredients, except the cheese, in a medium bowl and place in a 13 × 9-inch baking pan coated with cooking spray.

2 Bake, covered, for 50 minutes or until potatoes are tender. Remove from oven and sprinkle with cheese. Let stand, uncovered, for 5 minutes to absorb flavors.

1 (20-ounce) package refrigerated shredded hash browns (or **7 cups** frozen variety, thawed)

1$\frac{1}{2}$ **cups** frozen corn, thawed

$\frac{1}{2}$ (14-ounce) package frozen pepper stir fry, thawed

2 (4-ounce) cans chopped green chilies

1$\frac{1}{4}$ **cups** egg substitute

2 **tablespoons** canola oil

$\frac{1}{2}$ **teaspoon** dried oregano leaves

$\frac{3}{4}$ **teaspoon** salt

1 **cup** shredded reduced-fat sharp cheddar cheese

EXCHANGES / CHOICES
1$\frac{1}{2}$ Starch
1 Protein, lean
1 Fat

BASIC NUTRITIONAL VALUES

Calories	195	**Potassium**	385 mg
Calories from Fat	65	**Total Carbohydrate**	25 g
Total Fat	7.0 g	Dietary Fiber	3 g
Saturated Fat	2.1 g	Sugars	4 g
Trans Fat	0.0 g	**Protein**	9 g
Cholesterol	10 mg	**Phosphorus**	145 mg
Sodium	575 mg		

Hot Berry Bowls

4 cups fresh, or frozen and thawed, mixed berries
2 tablespoons sugar
$^1/_2$ **teaspoon** almond extract
$^3/_4$ **cup** low-fat granola, crumbled
2 cups plain nonfat Greek yogurt

1 Combine the berries, sugar, and almond extract in a microwave-safe bowl. Sprinkle with granola and cover.

2 Microwave for 5 minutes or until bubbly. Spoon into 6 individual dessert bowls and top with equal amounts of yogurt.

EXCHANGES / CHOICES
2 Carbohydrate

BASIC NUTRITIONAL VALUES

Calories	150	**Potassium**	260 mg
Calories from Fat	10	**Total Carbohydrate**	27 g
Total Fat	1.0 g	Dietary Fiber	4 g
Saturated Fat	0.1 g	Sugars	17 g
Trans Fat	0.0 g	**Protein**	10 g
Cholesterol	0 mg	**Phosphorus**	150 mg
Sodium	65 mg		

SERVES: 4
SERVING SIZE: 1 filled tortilla

1 Heat oil in a large nonstick skillet over medium heat. Cook peppers, onions, and paprika 8 minutes or until beginning to brown on edges. Pour the egg substitute over all and cook until set, about 1 minute, stirring gently.

2 Remove from heat, spoon equal amounts of the egg mixture, picante sauce, avocado, and cilantro on top of each tortilla. Serve with lime wedges, if desired.

1 **teaspoon** canola oil
1 **cup** chopped green bell pepper
1 **cup** chopped onion
$^1/_2$ **teaspoon** smoked paprika
1 **cup** egg substitute
$^1/_2$ **cup** picante sauce
1 **ripe** medium avocado, diced
$^1/_4$ **cup** chopped fresh cilantro
4 (8-inch) low-fat, low-carb flour tortillas
1 medium lime, quartered (optional)

COOK'S TIP: May fold edges over to be a breakfast wrap or serve with knife and fork to be an open-faced tortilla stack.

EXCHANGES / CHOICES
1 Starch
2 Vegetable
1 Protein, lean
1 Fat

BASIC NUTRITIONAL VALUES

Calories	215	**Potassium**	540 mg
Calories from Fat	80	**Total Carbohydrate**	28 g
Total Fat	9.0 g	Dietary Fiber	10 g
Saturated Fat	1.9 g	Sugars	5 g
Trans Fat	0.0 g	**Protein**	12 g
Cholesterol	0 mg	**Phosphorus**	130 mg
Sodium	570 mg		

Toaster Waffles and Strawberry-Almond Topping

SERVES: 4
SERVING SIZE: 1 waffle, $1/2$ cup berry mixture, and $1/4$ cup yogurt per serving

2 cups quartered strawberries
$1/2$ cup slivered almonds
$1\,1/2$ tablespoons pourable sugar substitute
$1/2$ teaspoon almond extract
4 whole-grain low-fat frozen waffles
1 cup nonfat plain Greek yogurt

1 Combine strawberries, almonds, sugar substitute, and extract in a medium bowl.

2 Toast waffles. Serve topped with equal amounts of the yogurt and strawberry mixture.

EXCHANGES / CHOICES	BASIC NUTRITIONAL VALUES			
1 Starch	Calories	215	Potassium	355 mg
$1/2$ Fruit	Calories from Fat	80	Total Carbohydrate	25 g
1 Protein, lean	Total Fat	9.0 g	Dietary Fiber	5 g
$1\,1/2$ Fat	Saturated Fat	0.8 g	Sugars	9 g
	Trans Fat	0.0 g	Protein	12 g
	Cholesterol	0 mg	Phosphorus	260 mg
	Sodium	220 mg		

Breakfast Berry Scooper Cake and Yogurt

Serves: 9
Serving Size: $2\frac{1}{2}$-inch square and $\frac{1}{3}$ cup yogurt per serving

1 cup all-purpose flour
7 tablespoons sugar, divided use
$\frac{1}{2}$ **teaspoon** baking powder
$\frac{1}{2}$ **teaspoon** baking soda
$\frac{1}{2}$ **teaspoon** ground cinnamon
$\frac{1}{8}$ **teaspoon** salt
$\frac{1}{2}$ **cup** nonfat buttermilk
1 large egg
3 tablespoons canola oil
$\frac{1}{2}$ **teaspoon** almond extract
1 (1-pound) bag frozen mixed berries
3 cups plain nonfat Greek yogurt

1 Preheat oven to 350°F. Meanwhile, combine the flour, all but 2 teaspoons of the sugar, baking powder, baking soda, cinnamon, salt, buttermilk, egg, oil, and extract in a medium bowl. Whisk together until smooth and pour into an 8-inch baking pan coated with cooking spray, top with the frozen berries.

2 Bake 1 hour or until browned and wooden pick inserted 2 inches from edge comes out clean. Remove from oven, place pan on cooling rack, and sprinkle with remaining sugar. Serve hot, warm, or room temperature with yogurt on the side.

Cook's Tip: If serving hot, use a spoon to remove. It will be a "loose" pudding cake texture. If serving warm, carefully cut into squares and use a flat spatula to remove; it will be a very moist pudding cake texture. If serving room temperature, cut into squares. Use a flat spatula to remove. It will be a firmer, but still very moist pudding cake texture.

EXCHANGES / CHOICES

2 Carbohydrate
1 Protein, lean
$\frac{1}{2}$ Fat

BASIC NUTRITIONAL VALUES

Calories	215	**Potassium**	180 mg
Calories from Fat	45	**Total Carbohydrate**	30 g
Total Fat	5.0 g	Dietary Fiber	2 g
Saturated Fat	0.5 g	Sugars	17 g
Trans Fat	0.0 g	**Protein**	11 g
Cholesterol	20 mg	**Phosphorus**	170 mg
Sodium	175 mg		

Cheese and Veggie Toasters

1 1/2 **tablespoons** light mayonnaise

1 1/2 **teaspoons** Dijon mustard

1 **teaspoon** dried oregano leaves

1/8 **teaspoon** dried pepper flakes

4 **ounces** multi-grain loaf bread, halved lengthwise and cut each in half crosswise

1/3 **cup** shredded reduced-fat Italian blend or Mexican blend cheese

1/2 **cup** diced green bell pepper

1/2 **cup** diced tomato

1. Preheat broiler. Meanwhile, stir together the mayonnaise, mustard, oregano, and pepper flakes in a small bowl, spread equal amounts on each baguette half. Place on baking sheet and sprinkle evenly with the cheese, peppers, and tomatoes.

2. Broil no closer than 5 inches away from heat source, for 2 minutes or until cheese has melted slightly and bread is browned on edges.

COOK'S TIP: This makes a super-quick lunch as well!

EXCHANGES / CHOICES

1 Starch
1 Protein, lean

BASIC NUTRITIONAL VALUES

Calories	125	**Potassium**	170 mg
Calories from Fat	35	**Total Carbohydrate**	16 g
Total Fat	4.0 g	Dietary Fiber	3 g
Saturated Fat	1.4 g	Sugars	3 g
Trans Fat	0.0 g	**Protein**	7 g
Cholesterol	5 mg	**Phosphorus**	150 mg
Sodium	285 mg		

LUNCH

Hearty Sausage and Rice Soup with Greens

SERVES: 4
SERVING SIZE: 1 1/2 cups

2 tablespoons extra virgin olive oil, divided use

6 ounces hot Italian chicken sausage, removed from casing

1 cup diced red bell pepper

1/2 cup quick-cooking brown rice

2 cups reduced-sodium chicken broth

1 cup water

1 cup frozen sliced carrots

4 ounces sliced mushrooms

2 cups packed chopped kale or spinach

1 Heat 1 teaspoon of the oil in a large saucepan over medium-high heat. Cook sausage and bell peppers 4 minutes or until sausage is browned, breaking up large pieces. Stir in rice, broth, water, carrots, and mushrooms. Bring to boil over high heat, reduce heat to medium low, cover, and cook 15 minutes or until carrots are tender,

2 Remove from heat, stir in kale and remaining oil, cover and cook 5 minutes or until kale is wilted.

EXCHANGES / CHOICES

1 Starch
2 Vegetable
1 Protein, lean
2 Fat

BASIC NUTRITIONAL VALUES

Calories	265	Potassium	625 mg
Calories from Fat	110	Total Carbohydrate	28 g
Total Fat	12.0 g	Dietary Fiber	4 g
Saturated Fat	2.2 g	Sugars	7 g
Trans Fat	0.0 g	Protein	13 g
Cholesterol	35 mg	Phosphorus	215 mg
Sodium	535 mg		

Sausage and Cabbage Soup

1 Heat oil in a Dutch oven over medium-high heat, brown the sausage, breaking up larger pieces. Add the remaining ingredients, except ketchup.

2 Bring to a boil, reduce to medium-low heat, cover, and simmer 15 minutes or until pasta is tender. Stir in ketchup.

1 teaspoon canola oil
6 ounces hot Italian chicken sausage, casings removed
4 cups coarsely chopped cabbage
2 cups chopped green bell pepper
1 cup frozen cut green beans
1 (14.5-ounce) can no-salt-added stewed tomatoes
2 ounces whole-grain or multigrain rotini pasta
3 1/2 cups water
1 tablespoon no-salt-added beef bouillon granules
1/4 teaspoon salt
1/3 cup ketchup

EXCHANGES / CHOICES
1/2 Starch
1/2 Carbohydrate
3 Vegetable
1 Fat

BASIC NUTRITIONAL VALUES

Calories	185	**Potassium**	875 mg
Calories from Fat	45	**Total Carbohydrate**	29 g
Total Fat	5.0 g	Dietary Fiber	6 g
Saturated Fat	1.1 g	Sugars	13 g
Trans Fat	0.0 g	**Protein**	11 g
Cholesterol	25 mg	**Phosphorus**	125 mg
Sodium	530 mg		

Grilled Tomato & Escarole Soup

4 medium tomatoes, halved crosswise
(1 pound total)
1 tablespoon extra-virgin olive oil
1 (16-ounce) can no-salt-added
garbanzo beans, rinsed and drained
2 cups vegetable broth, unsalted
2 tablespoons tomato paste
3 cups loosely packed escarole
(or spinach), coarsely chopped
¼ cup chopped fresh basil
2 teaspoons chopped fresh rosemary
2 teaspoons mild Louisiana hot sauce,
such as Frank's

1 Preheat grill to medium-high heat. Brush the tomato halves with the oil. Grill the tomatoes for 10 minutes or until tender, turning midway.

2 Combine the tomatoes, beans, broth, and tomato paste in a large saucepan. Bring to a boil, reduce heat to medium-low, cover, and cook 5 minutes. Stir in the remaining ingredients, breaking up larger pieces of tomato. Let stand 5 minutes to allow flavors to absorb.

EXCHANGES / CHOICES
1½ Starch
1 Vegetable
1 Fat

BASIC NUTRITIONAL VALUES

Calories	195	**Potassium**	675 mg
Calories from Fat	55	**Total Carbohydrate**	29 g
Total Fat	6.0 g	Dietary Fiber	8 g
Saturated Fat	0.7 g	Sugars	8 g
Trans Fat	0.0 g	**Protein**	8 g
Cholesterol	0 mg	**Phosphorus**	175 mg
Sodium	300 mg		

Chicken–White Bean Soup with Fresh Veggie Topper

Serves: 4

Serving Size: 1¼ cups soup and ⅔ cup topping per serving

1 Combine the soup ingredients in a large saucepan. Bring to a boil, reduce heat, and simmer, covered, 10 minutes or until pepper is tender. Remove from heat.

2 Combine the topping ingredients, except lime wedges, and spoon equal amounts on top of each serving of soup. Serve with lime wedges.

Cook's Tip: You can purchase pre-chopped onions, peppers, and tomatoes in the produce section as well as cooked diced chicken in the freezer section!

Soup

3 cups reduced-sodium chicken broth
2 cups cooked diced chicken breast meat
1 (15.8-ounce) can no-salt-added Great Northern beans, rinsed and drained
¾ cup diced green bell pepper or 1 medium poblano chili pepper, finely chopped
1 tablespoon chili powder
1½ teaspoons ground cumin

Topping

1 cup diced tomatoes
1 ripe medium avocado, diced
½ cup finely chopped green onion
½ cup chopped fresh cilantro
1 tablespoon extra virgin olive oil
⅛ teaspoon salt = 0.04 tsp tog
1 medium lime, cut in four wedges

EXCHANGES / CHOICES
1 Starch
2 Vegetable
3 Protein, lean
1½ Fat

BASIC NUTRITIONAL VALUES

Calories	325	Potassium	1010 mg 1042
Calories from Fat	110	Total Carbohydrate	25 g
Total Fat	12.0 g	Dietary Fiber	10 g
Saturated Fat	2.2 g	Sugars	4 g
Trans Fat	0.0 g	Protein	31 g 32
Cholesterol	60 mg	Phosphorus	350 mg 360
Sodium	560 mg 607		

Black Bean and Tomato Soup

Soup

2 (14.5-ounce) cans no-salt-added stewed tomatoes

1 (15-ounce) can no-salt-added black beans, rinsed and drained

2 (4.5-ounce) cans chopped mild green chilies

1 cup water

1 tablespoon chili powder

1 teaspoon ground cumin

1/8 teaspoon salt

Toppings

1/2 cup chopped fresh cilantro

2 ounces shredded reduced-fat cheddar cheese

1/2 cup fat-free sour cream

1 Combine all soup ingredients in a large saucepan. Bring to a boil over high heat, reduce heat to medium low, cover, and simmer 20 minutes or until thickened slightly. Remove from heat.

2 Top with equal amounts of the toppings.

EXCHANGES / CHOICES	BASIC NUTRITIONAL VALUES			
1 Starch	**Calories**	235	**Potassium**	940 mg
1/2 Milk, fat-free	Calories from Fat	40	**Total Carbohydrate**	41 g
4 Vegetable	**Total Fat**	4.5 g	Dietary Fiber	8 g
1/2 Fat	Saturated Fat	2.1 g	Sugars	16 g
	Trans Fat	0.0 g	**Protein**	13 g
	Cholesterol	10 mg	**Phosphorus**	270 mg
	Sodium	570 mg		

Tarragon Chicken, Garbanzo, and Kale Salad

1 Combine all ingredients, except spring greens, in a large bowl. Serve as is or on equal amounts of spring greens.

2 Serve immediately for peak flavors.

2 **cups** cooked diced chicken breast meat
1 (15-ounce) can no-salt-added garbanzo beans, rinsed and drained
½ **cup** diced red onion
1 **cup** finely chopped kale
2 **tablespoons** canola oil
1 **tablespoon** balsamic vinegar
2 **teaspoons** Dijon mustard
½ **teaspoon** dried tarragon leaves
¼ **teaspoon** salt
¼ **teaspoon** black pepper
1¼ **ounce** reduced-fat blue cheese or reduced-fat feta, crumbled
4 **cups** spring greens, optional

COOK'S TIP: If not serving immediately, add an additional 1 tablespoon vinegar to the recipe.

EXCHANGES / CHOICES
1 Starch
1 Vegetable
4 Protein, lean
1 Fat

BASIC NUTRITIONAL VALUES

Calories	340	**Potassium**	530 mg
Calories from Fat	115	**Total Carbohydrate**	24 g
Total Fat	13.0 g	Dietary Fiber	6 g
Saturated Fat	2.5 g	Sugars	6 g
Trans Fat	0.0 g	**Protein**	31 g
Cholesterol	65 mg	**Phosphorus**	335 mg
Sodium	390 mg		

Butter Lettuce Salad with Pears, Bacon, and Cilantro

SERVES: 4
SERVING SIZE: 2 cups

Salad

8 cups torn butter lettuce (1 head total)
¹/₂ cup thinly sliced red onion
(about **2 ounces** total) OR diced
³/₄ cup shelled edamame
1 firm medium pear, halved, cored,
and sliced
¹/₄ cup chopped fresh cilantro
8 cooked turkey bacon slices, chopped
1 ounce chopped walnuts

Dressing

2 tablespoons canola oil
3 tablespoons lemon juice
1 ¹/₂ tablespoons sugar
¹/₈ teaspoon dried pepper flakes
¹/₄ teaspoon salt

1 Combine salad ingredients in a large bowl.

2 Whisk together the dressing ingredients in a small bowl and toss with the salad ingredients.

EXCHANGES / CHOICES	BASIC NUTRITIONAL VALUES			
¹/₂ Fruit	**Calories**	270	**Potassium**	615 mg
¹/₂ Carbohydrate	Calories from Fat	160	**Total Carbohydrate**	21 g
1 Vegetable	**Total Fat**	18.0 g	Dietary Fiber	5 g
1 Protein, lean	Saturated Fat	2.3 g	Sugars	12 g
3 Fat	Trans Fat	0.1 g	**Protein**	11 g
	Cholesterol	25 mg	**Phosphorus**	185 mg
	Sodium	480 mg		

SERVES: 4
SERVING SIZE: 3 stuffed lettuce leaves

1 Combine salsa, mayonnaise, sour cream, and cumin in a medium bowl. Stir in the chicken, onion, and chili peppers.

2 Spoon equal amounts of the chicken mixture down the center of each lettuce leaf. Sprinkle evenly with the cilantro, cheese, and olives. Serve with lime wedges.

$^1/_3$ **cup** chunky medium salsa
$^1/_4$ **cup** light mayonnaise
$^1/_4$ **cup** fat-free sour cream
$^1/_2$ **teaspoon** ground cumin (optional)
2 cups cooked chopped chicken breast
$^1/_2$ **cup** diced red onion
1 medium poblano chili pepper, diced
12 large romaine lettuce leaves
$^1/_2$ **cup** chopped fresh cilantro
1 $^1/_2$ **ounces** shredded reduced-fat sharp cheddar cheese
1 (2.25-ounce) can sliced ripe olives, drained
1 medium lime, quartered

EXCHANGES / CHOICES

2 Vegetable
3 Protein, lean
1 $^1/_2$ Fat

BASIC NUTRITIONAL VALUES

Calories	255	**Potassium**	530 mg
Calories from Fat	100	**Total Carbohydrate**	13 g
Total Fat	11.0 g	Dietary Fiber	3 g
Saturated Fat	2.6 g	Sugars	5 g
Trans Fat	0.0 g	**Protein**	27 g
Cholesterol	70 mg	**Phosphorus**	275 mg
Sodium	505 mg		

White Bean and Pearl Couscous Main Salad

1 1/4 **cups** water

4 **ounces** uncooked whole-wheat Israeli pearl couscous or regular couscous

1/2 (15.8-ounce) **can** reduced-sodium Great Northern beans, rinsed and drained

1 medium cucumber, diced

1 **cup** grape tomatoes, quartered

1/2 **cup** diced red onion

2 1/2 **ounces** small pimiento-stuffed olives, coarsely chopped

2 **ounces** part-skim mozzarella cheese, diced

2 1/2 to 3 **tablespoons** cider vinegar

2 **tablespoons** extra virgin olive oil

1 **teaspoon** dried basil leaves

1 medium garlic clove, minced

1/4 **teaspoon** salt

1 Bring the water to a boil in a medium saucepan, add the couscous, cover, and cook on medium-low heat for 8–10 minutes or until tender. Drain in a fine-mesh sieve and run under cold water until cooled completely, shaking off excess liquid.

2 Place couscous in a medium bowl with the remaining ingredients and toss until well blended.

EXCHANGES / CHOICES

2 Starch
1 Vegetable
1 Protein, lean
1 1/2 Fat

BASIC NUTRITIONAL VALUES

Calories	295	**Potassium**	460 mg
Calories from Fat	110	**Total Carbohydrate**	37 g
Total Fat	12.0 g	Dietary Fiber	5 g
Saturated Fat	2.8 g	Sugars	4 g
Trans Fat	0.0 g	**Protein**	11 g
Cholesterol	10 mg	**Phosphorus**	180 mg
Sodium	540 mg		

Chicken Bulgur Salad with Raisins

1 Bring water to a boil in a medium saucepan. Add bulgur, reduce heat, cover, and cook on medium-low heat for 12 minutes. Drain in a fine-mesh sieve and run under cold water until completely cooled, shaking off excess liquid.

2 Place in a medium bowl and stir in the remaining ingredients.

COOK'S TIP: Let stand 15 minutes to allow flavors to absorb, if time allows.

2 **cups** water
$^1/_2$ **cup** quick-cooking bulgur
1 $^1/_2$ **cups** cooked chopped chicken breast
$^1/_2$ **cup** diced yellow bell pepper
$^1/_3$ **cup** diced red onion
$^1/_2$ **cup** raisins or golden raisins
1 **ounce** ($^1/_4$ **cup**) chopped walnuts
$^1/_2$ **cup** chopped fresh mint
2 **tablespoons** canola oil
2 **tablespoons** white balsamic vinegar
1 **teaspoon** pourable sugar substitute (optional)
1 $^1/_2$ **teaspoon** grated gingerroot
$^1/_2$ **teaspoon** salt
$^1/_8$ **teaspoon** dried pepper flakes

EXCHANGES / CHOICES	BASIC NUTRITIONAL VALUES			
1 Starch	**Calories**	340	**Potassium**	465 mg
1 Fruit	Calories from Fat	125	**Total Carbohydrate**	36 g
1 Vegetable	**Total Fat**	14.0 g	Dietary Fiber	6 g
3 Protein, lean	Saturated Fat	1.6 g	Sugars	14 g
1 Fat	Trans Fat	0.0 g	**Protein**	21 g
	Cholesterol	45 mg	**Phosphorus**	210 mg
	Sodium	340 mg		

Potato, Edamame, and Egg Salad

Serves: 5
Serving Size: 1 1/2 cups

6 **cups** water

1 **pound** red potatoes, unpeeled and cut into bite-size pieces

1 **cup** shelled edamame

4 hard-boiled eggs, chopped

1 **cup** sliced celery

1 **cup** diced red or green bell pepper

1/2 **cup** diced red onion

1/2 **cup** light mayonnaise

2 **tablespoons** cider vinegar

1 medium garlic clove, minced

2 **teaspoons** Dijon mustard

1 **tablespoon** dried dill

1/2 **teaspoon** salt

1 Bring water to boil in a large saucepan. Add the potatoes, return to a boil, reduce heat to medium-low, cover, and cook 7–8 minutes or until just tender when pierced with a fork.

2 Drain in a colander, run under cold water to cool quickly, and combine with the remaining ingredients in a large bowl.

COOK'S TIP: Try serving this with cucumber spears or on top of tomato slices for an extra taste of "fresh!"

EXCHANGES / CHOICES

1 1/2 Starch
1 Vegetable
1 Protein, medium fat
1 Fat

BASIC NUTRITIONAL VALUES

Calories	260	**Potassium**	705 mg
Calories from Fat	110	**Total Carbohydrate**	29 g
Total Fat	12.0 g	Dietary Fiber	5 g
Saturated Fat	2.3 g	Sugars	6 g
Trans Fat	0.1 g	**Protein**	11 g
Cholesterol	155 mg	**Phosphorus**	205 mg
Sodium	550 mg		

Asian Walnut Slaw with Pork

SERVES: 4
SERVING SIZE: 2 cups

1   Heat 1 teaspoon of the oil in a large skillet over medium-high heat. Cook the pork until slightly pink in center, stirring occasionally. Remove from heat and let cool.

2   Combine the pork with the remaining ingredients in a large bowl, except the walnuts. Toss until well blended. Sprinkle with the walnuts.

2 tablespoons canola oil, divided use
8 ounces boneless pork chops, trimmed of fat, cut into small bite-size pieces
1 (14-ounce) bag coleslaw or broccoli coleslaw
1 (8-ounce) can sliced water chestnuts, drained and thinly sliced
2 medium jalapeños, seeded and finely chopped
$^1/_2$ cup chopped fresh cilantro
2 tablespoons cider vinegar
2 tablespoons sugar
2 tablespoons light soy sauce
$^1/_4$ teaspoon salt
1 teaspoon grated ginger (optional)
1 ounce chopped walnuts

COOK'S TIP: If you have leftover cooked pork or chicken, replace the uncooked pork with 1 $^1/_2$ cups cooked diced pork or chicken and skip Step 1.

EXCHANGES / CHOICES	BASIC NUTRITIONAL VALUES			
$^1/_2$ Carbohydrate	**Calories**	280	**Potassium**	595 mg
3 Vegetable	Calories from Fat	145	**Total Carbohydrate**	21 g
1 Protein, lean	**Total Fat**	16.0 g	Dietary Fiber	5 g
3 Fat	Saturated Fat	24 g	Sugars	10 g
	Trans Fat	0.0 g	**Protein**	13 g
	Cholesterol	25 mg	**Phosphorus**	140 mg
	Sodium	475 mg		

Tabouleh Salad with Lemon and Flax

1 (5.25-ounce) box tabouleh
1/4 **cup** ground flax meal
1 **cup** diced cucumber
1 **cup** grape tomatoes, quartered
1/2 **cup** chopped fresh mint
1/2 **cup** chopped fresh parsley
4 medium green onions, finely chopped
2 **tablespoons** canola oil
Grated rind and juice from 1 medium
    lemon
2 **ounces** reduced-fat feta, crumbled

1 Prepare tabouleh according to package directions. Place in a medium bowl, cover, and refrigerate 30 minutes to cool.

2 Combine the cooled tabouleh mixture with the remaining ingredients.

EXCHANGES / CHOICES
2 Starch
1 Vegetable
2 Fat

BASIC NUTRITIONAL VALUES

Calories	250	**Potassium**	345 mg
Calories from Fat	100	**Total Carbohydrate**	36 g
Total Fat	11.0 g	Dietary Fiber	11 g
Saturated Fat	1.8 g	Sugars	4 g
Trans Fat	0.0 g	**Protein**	10 g
Cholesterol	5 mg	**Phosphorus**	115 mg
Sodium	550 mg		

Tacos in a Bowl

1 **teaspoon** canola oil

12 **ounces** extra-lean (90% lean) ground beef

$^1/_2$ **cup** mild salsa (lowest sodium possible)

1 **tablespoon** smoked paprika

6 **cups** shredded romaine lettuce

4 **ounces** baked corn tortilla chips, coarsely crumbled

$^1/_2$ **cup** finely chopped green or diced red onions

$^1/_2$ **cup** chopped fresh cilantro

1 (2.25-ounce) can sliced ripe olives, drained

$^1/_2$ **cup** fat-free sour cream

1 medium lime, cut in 4 wedges

1 Heat the oil in a large skillet over medium-high heat. Cook the beef until browned (draining any fat), stir in the salsa and paprika.

2 Place equal amounts of the lettuce in each of 4 shallow bowls. Spoon equal amounts of the chips into each bowl, top with the beef mixture and the remaining ingredients in the order listed.

EXCHANGES / CHOICES

1 $^1/_2$ Starch
$^1/_2$ Milk, fat-free
1 Vegetable
2 Protein, lean
1 Fat

BASIC NUTRITIONAL VALUES

Calories	330	**Potassium**	725 mg
Calories from Fat	115	**Total Carbohydrate**	34 g
Total Fat	13.0 g	Dietary Fiber	5 g
Saturated Fat	34 g	Sugars	4 g
Trans Fat	04 g	**Protein**	22 g
Cholesterol	55 mg	**Phosphorus**	305 mg
Sodium	445 mg		

Avocado BLT

1 ripe **medium** avocado, halved, pitted, and peeled
1 1/2 to **2 tablespoons** lemon juice
8 reduced-calorie whole-wheat bread, preferably toasted, divided use
1/4 **cup** chopped fresh cilantro
1 large tomato, cut into 8 thin slices
1/4 **teaspoon** black pepper
1/4 **cup** very thinly sliced red onion ~~? fresh~~
8 pre-cooked bacon slices   *? fresh*
4 medium romaine leaves

1 Mash the avocado with the lemon juice in a medium bowl and spread equal amounts on top of 4 of the bread slices.

2 Top with the remaining ingredients, except the bread slices, in the order listed. Top with the remaining bread slices. Cut in half, if desired.

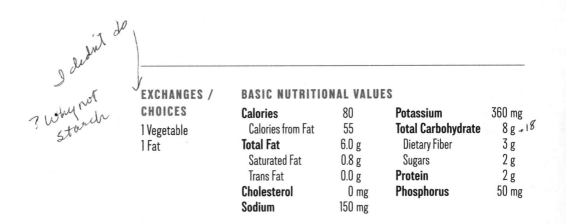

I didn't do
? why not starch

EXCHANGES / CHOICES	BASIC NUTRITIONAL VALUES			
1 Vegetable	**Calories**	80	**Potassium**	360 mg
1 Fat	Calories from Fat	55	**Total Carbohydrate**	8 g *·18*
	Total Fat	6.0 g	Dietary Fiber	3 g
	Saturated Fat	0.8 g	Sugars	2 g
	Trans Fat	0.0 g	**Protein**	2 g
	Cholesterol	0 mg	**Phosphorus**	50 mg
	Sodium	150 mg		

Turkey Sandwiches with Pesto, Mayonnaise, and Dried Cranberries

SERVES: 4
SERVING SIZE: 1 sandwich

1 Spread the mayonnaise on the bottom half of the bread. Top with the cranberries, onion, turkey, and spring greens.

2 Spread the pesto on the remaining top half of the bread. Place the bread on top of the spring greens, press down to adhere and cut into four slices.

$^1/_4$ **cup** light mayonnaise
8 ounces multi-grain Italian bread, cut in half lengthwise
2 tablespoons reduced-sugar dried cranberries
2 ounces very thinly sliced red onion ($^1/_2$ **cup**)
1$^1/_3$ cups cooked diced turkey or chicken breast meat
2 ounces (2 cups) packed spring greens
$^1/_4$ **cup** prepared pesto

COOK'S TIP: This is a scrumptious way to use your leftover turkey from the holidays . . . or anytime!

EXCHANGES / CHOICES	BASIC NUTRITIONAL VALUES			
1 $^1/_2$ Starch	**Calories**	315	**Potassium**	335 mg
$^1/_2$ Carbohydrate	Calories from Fat	100	**Total Carbohydrate**	33 g
3 Protein, lean	**Total Fat**	11.0 g	Dietary Fiber	6 g
1 Fat	Saturated Fat	1.9 g	Sugars	7 g
	Trans Fat	0.0 g	**Protein**	23 g
	Cholesterol	40 mg	**Phosphorus**	250 mg
	Sodium	560 mg		

Grilled Chicken Sandwich with Olive Arugula Topping

SERVES: 4
SERVING SIZE: 1 sandwich

Sandwich

4 (4-ounce) boneless chicken breast thin cutlets, rinsed and patted dry
Cooking spray
1 teaspoon dried basil leaves
1/2 teaspoon onion powder
1/8 teaspoon dried pepper flakes
8 ounces multi-grain Italian bread, cut in half lengthwise

Topping

2 cups packed arugula or spring greens
1/4 cup diced red onion
16 pitted kalamata olives, coarsely chopped
1 1/2 tablespoons extra-virgin olive oil
1 to 1 1/2 tablespoons red wine vinegar

1 Heat a large skillet over medium-high heat. Coat chicken with cooking spray and sprinkle with the basil, onion powder, and pepper flakes. Cook 5 minutes on each side or until no longer pink in center.

2 Meanwhile, combine the topping ingredients in a medium bowl. Place the chicken on bottom half of the bread, top with the arugula mixture, top with remaining bread, and cut into four sections.

EXCHANGES / CHOICES	BASIC NUTRITIONAL VALUES			
2 Starch	**Calories**	365	**Potassium**	405 mg
4 Protein, lean	Calories from Fat	125	**Total Carbohydrate**	27 g
1 Fat	**Total Fat**	14.0 g (13.1)	Dietary Fiber	5 g
	Saturated Fat	2.3 g	Sugars	4 g
	Trans Fat	0.0 g	**Protein**	32 g
	Cholesterol	65 mg	**Phosphorus**	315 mg
	Sodium	420 mg 441		

Serves: 4
Serving Size: 1 tortilla, $^1/_2$ cup lettuce, and $^1/_2$ cup egg mixture per serving

Egg and Veggie Hummus Wraps

1 Combine the eggs, cucumbers, onions, olives, and basil in a medium bowl.

2 Spread 3 tablespoons hummus on each tortilla, top with $^1/_2$ cup of the lettuce, and spoon equal amounts of the egg mixture down the center of each lettuce leaf. Squeeze lemon juice evenly over all. Fold edges over.

2 hard-boiled eggs, chopped
$^1/_2$ **cup** diced cucumber
$^1/_3$ **cup** diced red onion
12 pitted kalamata olives, coarsely chopped
$^1/_4$ **cup** chopped fresh basil
$^3/_4$ **cup** prepared hummus
4 low-carb, high-fiber tortillas, such as La Tortilla Factory, Garlic Herb variety
2 **cups** shredded romaine lettuce
1 medium lemon, quartered (optional)

Cook's Tip: No need to spend time boiling and cooling eggs, you can purchase cooked and peeled eggs in your deli or dairy aisle in your supermarket.

EXCHANGES / CHOICES	BASIC NUTRITIONAL VALUES			
1 Starch	Calories	195	Potassium	270 mg
1 Vegetable	Calories from Fat	100	**Total Carbohydrate**	20 g
1 Protein, lean	**Total Fat**	11.0 g	Dietary Fiber	10 g
1 $^1/_2$ Fat	Saturated Fat	1.7 g	Sugars	4 g
	Trans Fat	0.0 g	**Protein**	12 g
	Cholesterol	95 mg	**Phosphorus**	185 mg
	Sodium	485 mg		

Smoky Sloppy Joes

SERVES: 8
SERVING SIZE: 1/2 cup beef mixture and
1 hamburger bun per serving

1 teaspoon canola oil
1 pound extra-lean (90% lean) ground beef
1 cup diced onions
1 cup diced green bell pepper
1 (14.5-ounce) can no-salt-added stewed tomatoes
1 tablespoon sugar
2 teaspoons smoked paprika
1 tablespoon Worcestershire sauce
2 teaspoons cider vinegar
1/4 teaspoon ground allspice
1/2 teaspoon salt
1/4 teaspoon black pepper
8 whole-wheat hamburger buns

1 Heat the oil in a large skillet over medium-high heat. Brown the beef, stirring occasionally. Drain any fat from beef, and stir in the remaining ingredients, except the buns. Bring to a boil over medium-high heat, reduce heat to medium-low, cover, and cook for 15 minutes or until vegetables are tender.

2 Remove the lid and bring to a boil over medium-high heat. Boil 3–4 minutes or until slightly thickened. Serve with hamburger buns.

EXCHANGES / CHOICES

1 1/2 Starch
1 Vegetable
2 Protein, lean
1/2 Fat

BASIC NUTRITIONAL VALUES

Calories	245	230	Potassium	495 mg
Calories from Fat	65		Total Carbohydrate	31 g 19.7
Total Fat	7.0 g	8.8	Dietary Fiber	5 g
Saturated Fat	2.3 g		Sugars	10 g
Trans Fat	0.3 g		Protein	16 g 19.2
Cholesterol	35 mg		Phosphorus	215 mg
Sodium	395 mg			

Artichoke-Parmesan on Crusty Bread Halves

SERVES: 6
SERVING SIZE: 2 sandwich halves with $1/2$ cup filling

12 ounces multigrain Italian or French bread, cut in half lengthwise and cut each half into 6 pieces (making 12 pieces total)
$1/2$ of a 14-ounce can quartered artichokes, drained and chopped
6 ounces fat-free cream cheese
$1/3$ **cup** grated Parmesan cheese
2 tablespoons extra virgin olive oil
$1/3$ **cup** chopped fresh basil
1 medium garlic clove, minced
$1/8$ **teaspoon** salt
1 cup grape tomatoes, diced

1 Arrange the bread slices on a baking sheet in a single layer, place in oven, and turn oven on to 350°F. (No need to preheat oven.) Bake 8 minutes, turning midway. Remove from oven.

2 Meanwhile, combine remaining ingredients, except the tomatoes, in a medium bowl. Spoon equal amounts (2 tablespoons) on each bread slice and sprinkle evenly with the tomatoes.

COOK'S TIP: To serve as an appetizer, cut each bread slice $1/4$-inch thick and cut each in half, making 24 pieces total.

EXCHANGES / CHOICES	BASIC NUTRITIONAL VALUES			
1 Starch	**Calories**	125	**Potassium**	175 mg
1 Fat	Calories from Fat	35	**Total Carbohydrate**	15 g
	Total Fat	4.0 g	Dietary Fiber	3 g
	Saturated Fat	0.9 g	Sugars	3 g
	Trans Fat	0.0 g	**Protein**	7 g
	Cholesterol	5 mg	**Phosphorus**	165 mg
	Sodium	295 mg		

Skillet Tortilla Pizza

1 (10-inch) spinach flour tortilla
$^1/_4$ **cup** pizza sauce
$^1/_8$ **teaspoon** dried pepper flakes
   (optional)
$^1/_2$ **ounce** sliced turkey pepperoni, cut in
   half or **1 ounce** extra-lean diced ham
$^1/_4$ **cup** thinly sliced red onion
$^1/_4$ **cup** thinly sliced green bell pepper
$^1/_4$ **cup** chopped fresh basil
1 ounce shredded part-skim mozzarella

1 Coat both sides of the tortilla with cooking spray. Heat a large nonstick skillet over medium heat, cook tortilla 2 minutes.

2 Turn tortilla over. Using back of a spoon, spread the sauce evenly over all and sprinkle with remaining ingredients in order listed. Cover and cook 2 minutes or until cheese has melted. Remove and let stand 1 minute to allow the tortilla to become crisp. Cut into 4 wedges.

EXCHANGES / CHOICES	BASIC NUTRITIONAL VALUES			
1 Starch	**Calories**	95	**Potassium**	140 mg
$^1/_2$ Fat	Calories from Fat	30	**Total Carbohydrate**	12 g
	Total Fat	3.5 g	Dietary Fiber	1 g
	Saturated Fat	1.3 g	Sugars	2 g
	Trans Fat	0.1 g	**Protein**	5 g
	Cholesterol	10 mg	**Phosphorus**	90 mg
	Sodium	290 mg		

SERVES: 4
SERVING SIZE: 1/2 cup dip and 1 ounce chips or
8 pita wedges per serving

Greek Layered Bean Dip Bowls with Rice Chips

1 In a small bowl, combine the refried beans, yogurt, and garlic. Spoon into the bottom of a small shallow bowl. Top with remaining ingredients, except the rice chips, in the order listed.

2 To serve, spoon onto rice chips or pita wedges.

1/2 (16-ounce) can fat-free refried beans
1/2 cup nonfat plain Greek yogurt
1 medium garlic clove, minced
2 ounces diced plum tomatoes
1/2 cup diced cucumber
2 tablespoons chopped fresh basil
1 ounce reduced-fat feta cheese, crumbled
8 pitted kalamata olives, chopped
4 ounces rice chips, sea salt variety, such as Lundberg's or 2 pita bread rounds, cut in half to make 4 rounds and each cut into 8 wedges

EXCHANGES / CHOICES

2 Starch
1 Protein, lean
1 Fat

BASIC NUTRITIONAL VALUES

Calories	250	**Potassium**	425 mg
Calories from Fat	80	**Total Carbohydrate**	33 g
Total Fat	9.0 g	Dietary Fiber	4 g
Saturated Fat	1.2 g	Sugars	5 g
Trans Fat	0.0 g	**Protein**	10 g
Cholesterol	5 mg	**Phosphorus**	240 mg
Sodium	520 mg		

Pimiento Cheese Lunch Cracker Stacks

SERVES: 4
SERVING SIZE: 3 tablespoons cheese mixture, $^1/_4$ cup hummus, 2 apple slices, and 2 crisp breads per serving

1 (4-ounce) jar diced pimiento, well drained

1 $^1/_2$ **ounces** shredded reduced-fat sharp cheddar cheese

2 **tablespoons** light mayonnaise

2 **tablespoons** fat-free sour cream

1 **teaspoon** Dijon mustard

1 **teaspoon** mild Louisiana hot sauce, such as Frank's

1 **cup** prepared hummus

8 **pieces** high-fiber crisp breads

2 medium apples, cut in half then sliced

1 Combine the pimiento, cheese, mayonnaise, sour cream, mustard, and hot sauce in a medium bowl.

2 Spread 2 tablespoons of the hummus on each crisp bread and top with 1 $^1/_2$ tablespoons of the pimiento mixture and apple slices.

EXCHANGES / CHOICES	BASIC NUTRITIONAL VALUES			
2 $^1/_2$ Carbohydrate	**Calories**	260	**Potassium**	380 mg
1 Protein, lean	Calories from Fat	90	**Total Carbohydrate**	36 g
1 Fat	**Total Fat**	10.0 g	Dietary Fiber	9 g
	Saturated Fat	2.4 g	Sugars	15 g
	Trans Fat	0.0 g	**Protein**	10 g
	Cholesterol	10 mg	**Phosphorus**	235 mg
	Sodium	580 mg		

APPETIZERS, SNACKS

Lemon-Dill Yogurt Dip

1 cup plain nonfat Greek yogurt
1 tablespoon dried dill
1 medium garlic clove, minced
1/4 teaspoon salt
1 tablespoon extra virgin olive oil
2 teaspoons grated lemon zest

1 Whisk together the yogurt, dill, garlic, and salt in a small shallow bowl.

2 Drizzle the oil evenly over the top and sprinkle with the lemon zest.

COOK'S TIP: May serve with veggies, such as celery, cucumber, squash slices, carrot sticks, or grape tomatoes pierced with wooden picks.

EXCHANGES / CHOICES
1/2 Milk, fat-free
1/2 Fat

BASIC NUTRITIONAL VALUES

Calories	65	**Potassium**	110 mg
Calories from Fat	30	**Total Carbohydrate**	3 g
Total Fat	3.5 g	Dietary Fiber	0 g
Saturated Fat	0.5 g	Sugars	2 g
Trans Fat	0.0 g	**Protein**	6 g
Cholesterol	0 mg	**Phosphorus**	80 mg
Sodium	170 mg		

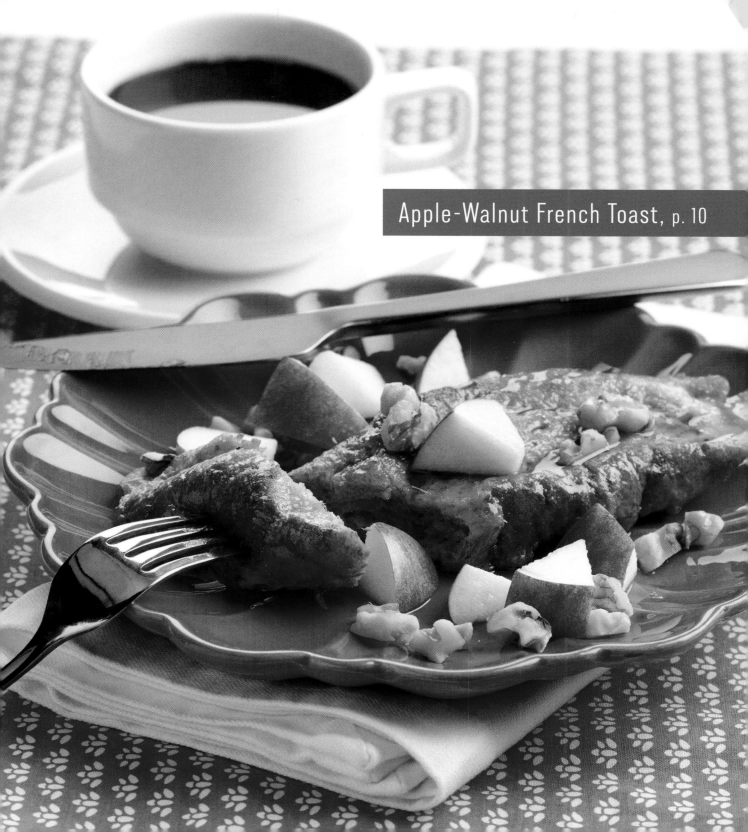

Apple-Walnut French Toast, p. 10

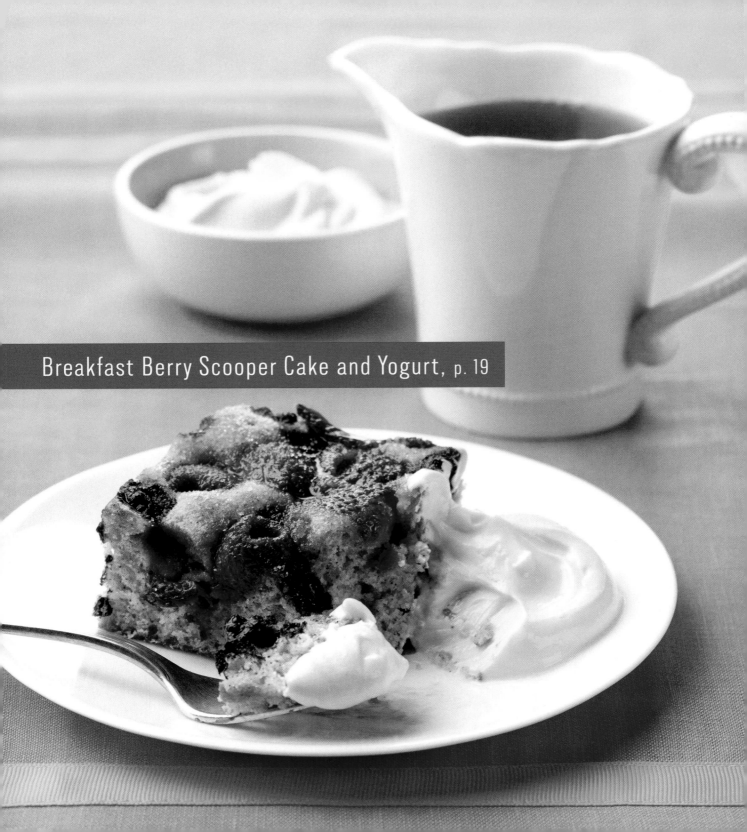

Breakfast Berry Scooper Cake and Yogurt, p. 19

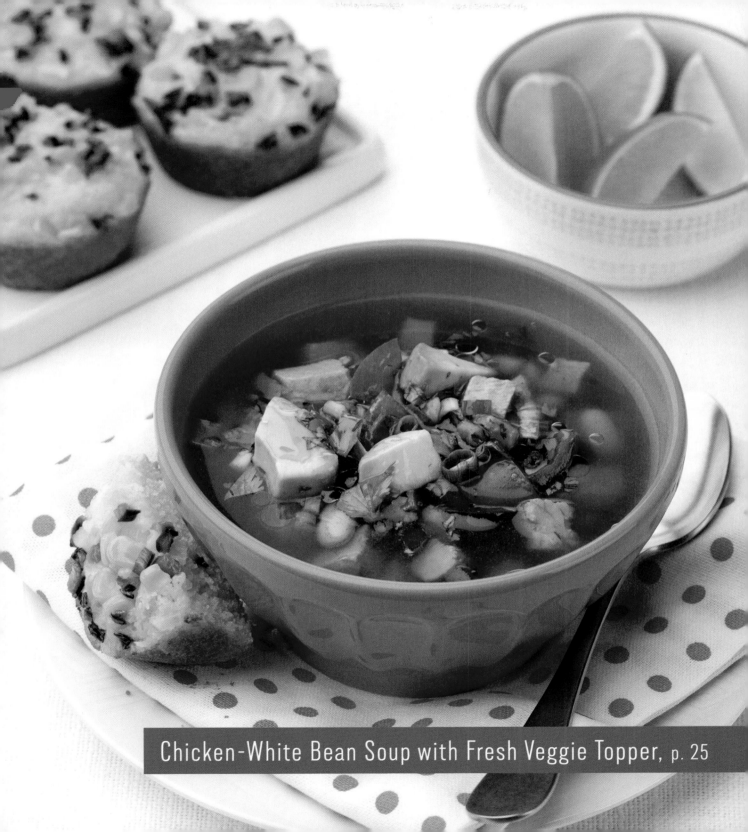

Chicken-White Bean Soup with Fresh Veggie Topper, p. 25

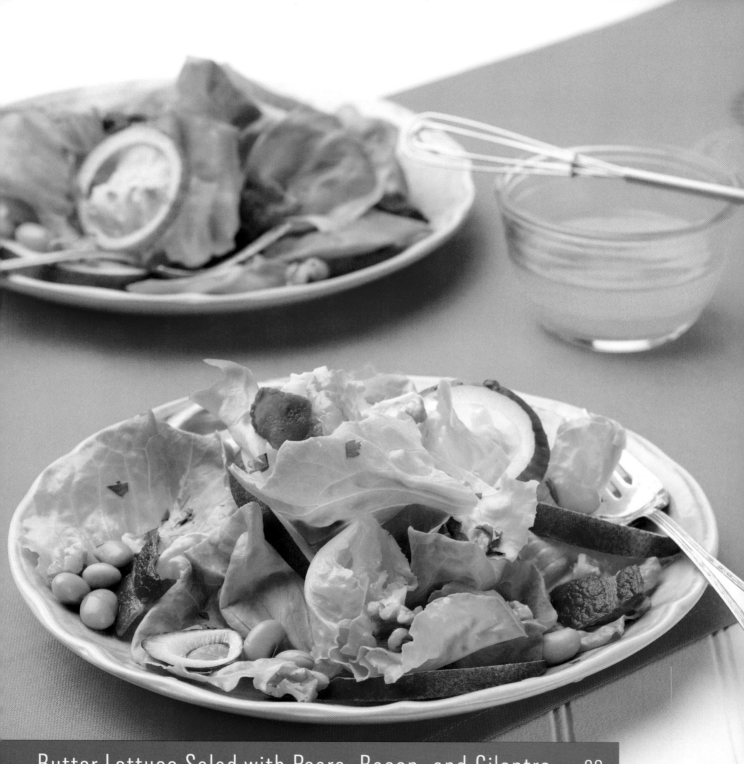

Butter Lettuce Salad with Pears, Bacon, and Cilantro, p. 28

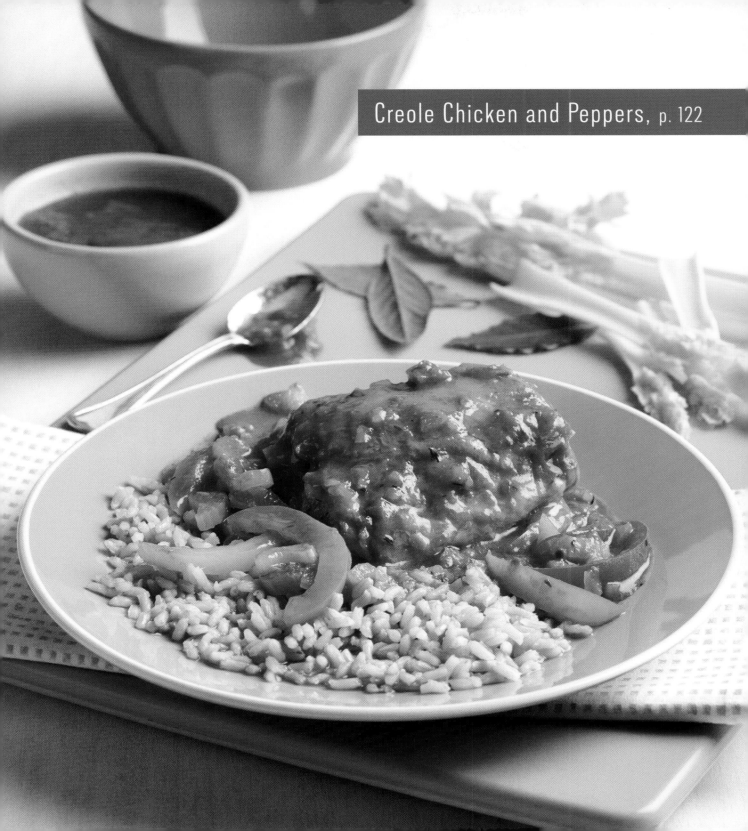

Creole Chicken and Peppers, p. 122

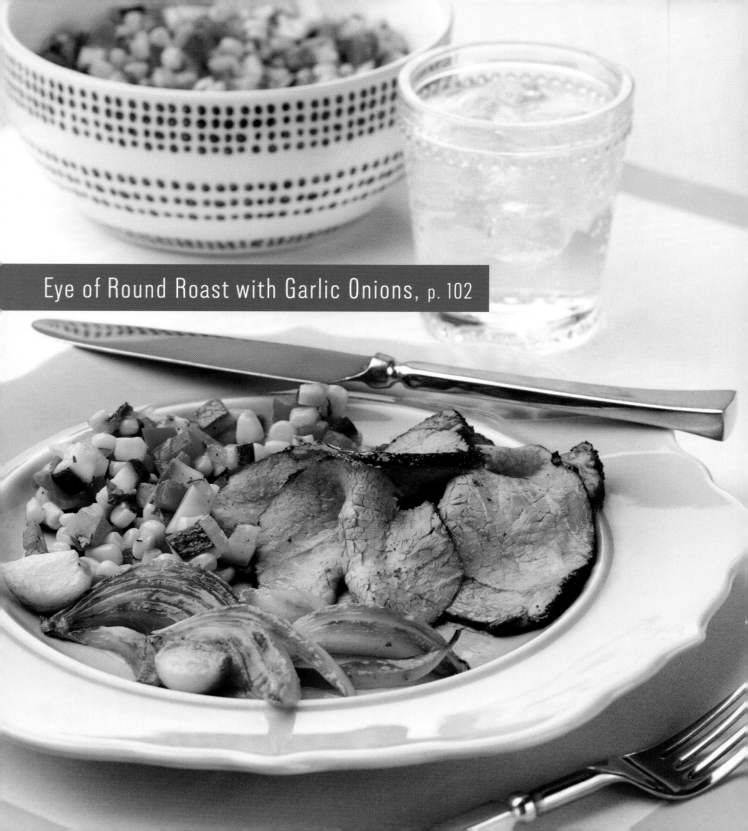

Eye of Round Roast with Garlic Onions, p. 102

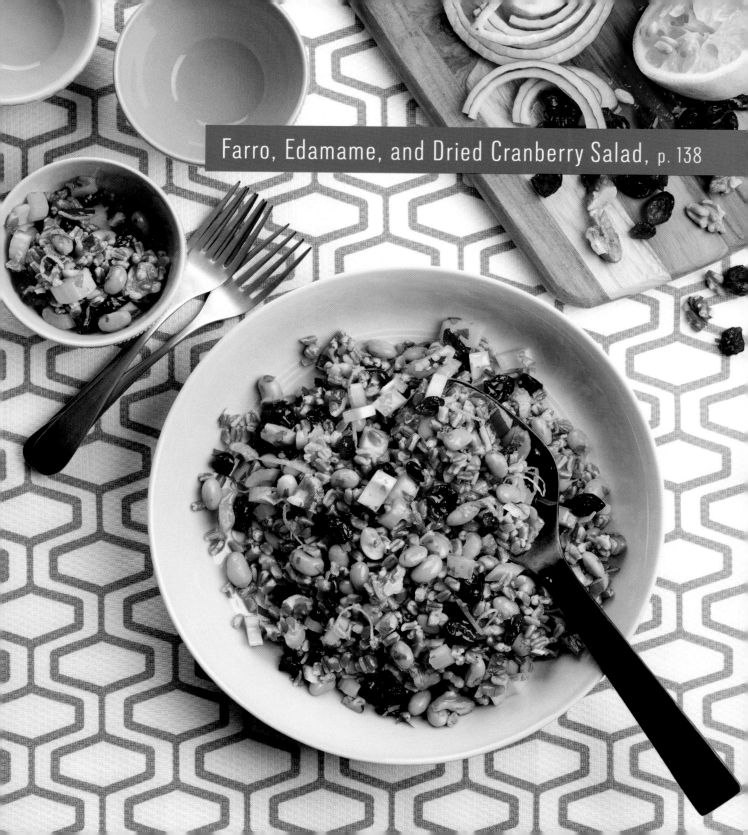

Farro, Edamame, and Dried Cranberry Salad, p. 138

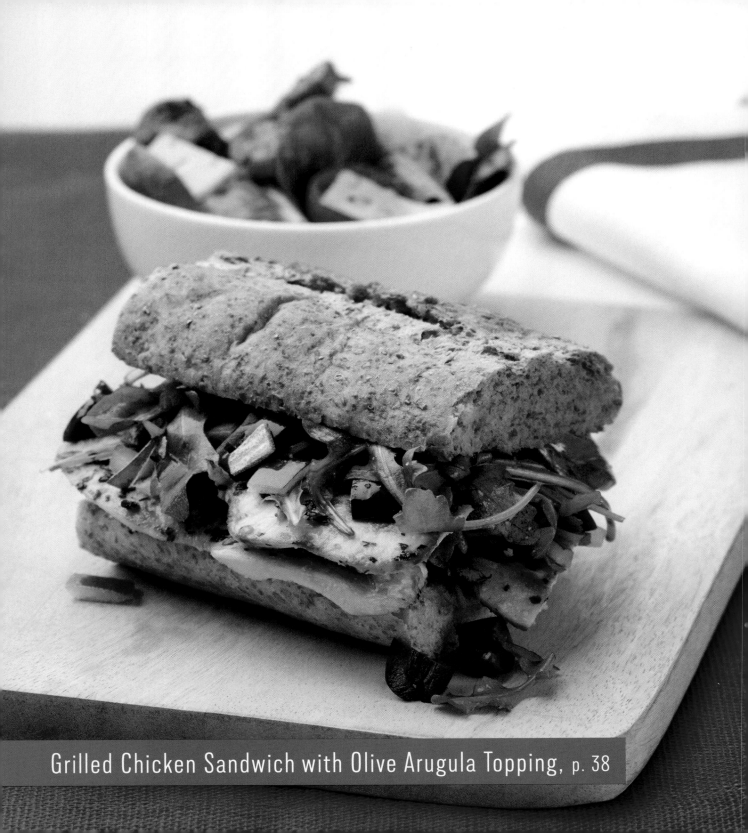

Grilled Chicken Sandwich with Olive Arugula Topping, p. 38

Lemon-Minted Hummus

SERVES: 6
SERVING SIZE: 1/4 cup

1 Place beans, water, lemon juice, garlic, oil, cumin, salt, and cayenne in a blender and purée 1 minute or until smooth.

2 Spoon into a shallow bowl and sprinkle evenly with the mint and lemon rind.

1 (15-ounce) can no-salt-added garbanzo beans, rinsed and drained
1/3 cup water
Grated rind and juice of 1 medium lemon
1 to 2 medium garlic cloves, peeled only
2 tablespoons extra virgin olive oil
1/2 teaspoon ground cumin
1/2 teaspoon salt
1/8 teaspoon cayenne pepper
1/4 cup chopped fresh mint

COOK'S TIP: May serve with raw veggies, such as bell pepper strips, cucumber slices, and celery sticks.

EXCHANGES / CHOICES
1 Starch
1 Fat

BASIC NUTRITIONAL VALUES

Calories	120	**Potassium**	165 mg
Calories from Fat	55	**Total Carbohydrate**	14 g
Total Fat	6.0 g	Dietary Fiber	4 g
Saturated Fat	0.8 g	Sugars	3 g
Trans Fat	0.0 g	**Protein**	4 g
Cholesterol	0 mg	**Phosphorus**	80 mg
Sodium	200 mg		

Whirled Fresh Lime, Avocado, and Cilantro

SERVES: 8
SERVING SIZE: 2 tablespoons

1 ripe medium avocado, peeled
  and pitted
$^1/_2$ **cup** chopped fresh cilantro
$^1/_4$ **cup** fat-free sour cream
$^1/_4$ **cup** light mayonnaise
1 medium garlic clove, minced
2 tablespoons lime juice
2 teaspoons mild Louisiana hot sauce,
  such as Frank's
$^1/_4$ **teaspoon** salt

1 Combine all ingredients in a blender and purée
until smooth.

COOK'S TIP: Serve as a spread for wraps and sandwiches, a dip for fresh veggies, or a topper for grilled fish or chicken.

EXCHANGES / CHOICES	BASIC NUTRITIONAL VALUES			
1 Fat	**Calories**	60	**Potassium**	115 mg
	Calories from Fat	40	**Total Carbohydrate**	4 g
	Total Fat	4.5 g	Dietary Fiber	1 g
	Saturated Fat	0.7 g	Sugars	1 g
	Trans Fat	0.0 g	**Protein**	1 g
	Cholesterol	0 mg	**Phosphorus**	20 mg
	Sodium	205 mg		

Creamy Eggplant-Garbanzo Dip

SERVES: 8
SERVING SIZE: ¼ cup

1 Preheat oven to 375°F. Meanwhile, coat both sides of the eggplant halves with cooking spray and place, cut side down, on a foil-lined baking sheet. Bake 20–22 minutes or until tender.

2 Turn eggplant over, scoop out the "meat" of the eggplant. To remove the "meat" of the hot eggplant easily, hold the stem end with a fork to keep the eggplant in place. With your other hand, use a tablespoon to scrape out the "meat" onto the foil-lined baking sheet. Discard the skins, pull up the ends of the foil, and slide the eggplant and its juices into the blender with all other ingredients. Purée until smooth. Serve warm or chilled.

COOK'S TIP: May serve with pita chips or fresh veggies, such as celery, carrots, cucumber, zucchini rounds, or grape tomatoes. May also serve as a sandwich or wrap spread. Freeze remaining garbanzo beans for a later use.

1 medium eggplant (about 1¼ pounds), pierced in several areas, cut in half lengthwise
½ (15-ounce) can garbanzo beans, rinsed and drained
¼ **cup** extra virgin olive oil
2 tablespoons lemon juice
2 medium garlic cloves, peeled
1 teaspoon smoked paprika
¾ **teaspoon** salt
½ **teaspoon** ground cumin

EXCHANGES / CHOICES
½ Carbohydrate
1½ Fat

BASIC NUTRITIONAL VALUES

Calories	105	**Potassium**	125 mg
Calories from Fat	65	**Total Carbohydrate**	10 g
Total Fat	7.0 g	Dietary Fiber	3 g
Saturated Fat	1.0 g	Sugars	3 g
Trans Fat	0.0 g	**Protein**	2 g
Cholesterol	0 mg	**Phosphorus**	35 mg
Sodium	245 mg		

Roasted Pepper & Olive Veggie Yogurt Dip

SERVES: 4
SERVING SIZE: $^1/_3$ cup

1 cup nonfat plain Greek yogurt

1 tablespoon extra virgin olive oil

2 tablespoons finely chopped fresh basil

12 pitted kalamata olives, finely chopped

2 tablespoons finely chopped roasted red pepper

1 Spoon yogurt in a small shallow bowl. Drizzle the oil evenly on top.

2 Sprinkle evenly with the remaining ingredients in the order listed. Serve with raw vegetables, such as cucumbers, yellow squash, celery, carrots, or cauliflower.

EXCHANGES / CHOICES

$^1/_2$ Milk, fat-free
1 Fat

BASIC NUTRITIONAL VALUES

Calories	90	**Potassium**	100 mg
Calories from Fat	55	**Total Carbohydrate**	3 g
Total Fat	6.0 g	Dietary Fiber	0 g
Saturated Fat	0.7 g	Sugars	3 g
Trans Fat	0.0 g	**Protein**	6 g
Cholesterol	0 mg	**Phosphorus**	80 mg
Sodium	130 mg		

Sweet Spiced Peanut Butter Dip

SERVES: 4

SERVING SIZE: 3 tablespoons dip and $^1/_2$ cup apple slices per serving

1. Combine all ingredients, except the apple slices, in a small microwave-safe bowl. Microwave on high setting for 1 minute, whisk together until well blended.

2. Serve with apple slices for dipping

$^1/_4$ **cup** reduced-fat peanut butter
$^1/_4$ **cup** fat-free cream cheese
$^1/_4$ **cup** fat-free milk
1 $^1/_2$ **tablespoons** sugar substitute
$^1/_4$ **teaspoon** ground cinnamon
2 **cups** tart apple slices, such as Granny Smith

COOK'S TIP: May replace apple slices with firm pear slices.

EXCHANGES / CHOICES	BASIC NUTRITIONAL VALUES			
$^1/_2$ Fruit	**Calories**	145	**Potassium**	225 mg
$^1/_2$ Carbohydrate	Calories from Fat	55	**Total Carbohydrate**	19 g
1 Protein, medium fat	**Total Fat**	6.0 g	Dietary Fiber	2 g
	Saturated Fat	1.1 g	Sugars	10 g
	Trans Fat	0.0 g	**Protein**	5 g
	Cholesterol	0 mg	**Phosphorus**	105 mg
	Sodium	125 mg		

Cinnamon Sweet Fruit Skewers

32 whole medium strawberries, stemmed

16 canned pineapple chunks packed in own juice, drained

16 seedless red or green grapes

8 (6-inch) bamboo skewers

1 ½ tablespoons pourable sugar substitute

½ teaspoon ground cinnamon

1 Thread alternating 2 strawberries, 1 pineapple chunk, and 1 grape per skewer. Repeat with remaining fruit and skewers.

2 At time of serving, combine the sugar substitute and cinnamon in a small bowl and sprinkle evenly over all.

COOK'S TIP: If not serving immediately, cover the skewers and refrigerate until needed. Sprinkle with cinnamon mixture at time of serving for peak flavors and texture. This makes a fun salad (as well as a snack) for kids of all ages, too.

EXCHANGES / CHOICES
1 Fruit

BASIC NUTRITIONAL VALUES

Calories	65	**Potassium**	225 mg
Calories from Fat	0	**Total Carbohydrate**	17 g
Total Fat	0.0 g	Dietary Fiber	3 g
Saturated Fat	0.0 g	Sugars	13 g
Trans Fat	0.0 g	**Protein**	1 g
Cholesterol	0 mg	**Phosphorus**	30 mg
Sodium	0 mg		

Caramelized Onion and Goat Cheese Phyllo Bites

SERVES: 5
SERVING SIZE: 3 shells

1 Heat the oil in a large skillet over medium-high heat. Cook the onions, fruit spread, and pepper flakes for 8–10 minutes or until richly browned, stirring frequently. Cool completely.

2 Combine the cheeses in a small bowl and spoon equal amounts of the cheese (1 teaspoon) in each phyllo shell. Top with equal amounts (about 2 slightly rounded teaspoons) of the onion mixture.

2 teaspoons canola oil
1 1/2 cups diced red onion
2 tablespoons strawberry fruit spread
1/8 teaspoon dried pepper flakes
1 ounce goat cheese or goat cheese with honey
1 1/2 ounces fat-free cream cheese
15 mini phyllo shells

COOK'S TIP: Serve onion mixture warm or at room temperature.

EXCHANGES / CHOICES

1 Carbohydrate
1 1/2 Fat

BASIC NUTRITIONAL VALUES

Calories	135	**Potassium**	110 mg
Calories from Fat	65	**Total Carbohydrate**	15 g
Total Fat	7.0 g	Dietary Fiber	1 g
Saturated Fat	1.4 g	Sugars	6 g
Trans Fat	0.0 g	**Protein**	3 g
Cholesterol	5 mg	**Phosphorus**	90 mg
Sodium	125 mg		

Pepperoni Mozzarella Pita Crisps

Serves: 4
Serving Size: about 7 pieces per serving

3 **ounces** pita chips
$^1/_2$ **cup** finely chopped red bell pepper
$^1/_2$ (4.25-ounce) can chopped (not sliced) ripe olives
$^1/_2$ **ounce** regular turkey pepperoni, chopped
$^3/_4$ **ounce** finely shredded part-skim mozzarella
1 $^1/_2$ **teaspoons** dried oregano leaves
$^1/_8$ **teaspoon** dried pepper flakes

1 Preheat oven to 400°F. Place pita wedges in a single layer in a 13 × 9-inch baking pan.

2 Combine the remaining ingredients in a medium bowl. Sprinkle the mixture on top of the pita wedges and bake 4 minutes or until cheese has melted slightly. Serve immediately for peak flavor and texture.

EXCHANGES / CHOICES

1 Starch
1 $^1/_2$ Fat

BASIC NUTRITIONAL VALUES

Calories	150	**Potassium**	100 mg
Calories from Fat	65	**Total Carbohydrate**	17 g
Total Fat	7.0 g	Dietary Fiber	2 g
Saturated Fat	1.2 g	Sugars	2 g
Trans Fat	0.0 g	**Protein**	5 g
Cholesterol	10 mg	**Phosphorus**	80 mg
Sodium	405 mg		

SERVES: 5
SERVING SIZE: 5 "cups" per serving

1 Preheat oven to 400°F. Arrange the tortilla cups in a single layer on a large baking sheet. Combine the remaining ingredients, except the cheese and sour cream, in a medium bowl. Gently stir in the cheese. Fill equal amounts in each of the tortilla "cups."

2 Bake 4 minutes or until the cheese is melted. Serve topped with ¼ teaspoon sour cream on each, if desired.

30 baked corn tortilla scoop-style chips, about 2 ounces total
³/₄ cup finely chopped green bell peppers
³/₄ finely chopped tomatoes, preferably grape tomatoes
¹/₃ cup chopped fresh cilantro
1 teaspoon dried oregano leaves
³/₄ teaspoon ground cumin
¹/₈ teaspoon dried red pepper flakes
¹/₄ teaspoon salt
2 ounces finely shredded reduced-fat sharp cheddar cheese or part-skim mozzarella cheese
¹/₄ cup fat-free sour cream (optional)

EXCHANGES / CHOICES
½ Starch
1 Fat

BASIC NUTRITIONAL VALUES

Calories	85	**Potassium**	135 mg
Calories from Fat	40	**Total Carbohydrate**	10 g
Total Fat	4.5 g	Dietary Fiber	1 g
Saturated Fat	1.4 g	Sugars	1 g
Trans Fat	0.0 g	**Protein**	4 g
Cholesterol	5 mg	**Phosphorus**	85 mg
Sodium	200 mg		

Mini Garlic Cheese Crostini

4 ounces multigrain baguette-style bread, cut into ⅛-inch thick slices (16 slices total)
2 tablespoons light mayonnaise
½ medium garlic clove, minced
¼ teaspoon Dijon mustard
2 tablespoons finely chopped fresh basil
1 ounce finely shredded part-skim mozzarella
1½ tablespoons grated Parmesan cheese

1 Arrange the bread slices on a baking sheet in a single layer, place in oven, and turn oven on 400°F (no need to preheat oven). Bake 5 minutes, turning midway. Remove from oven.

2 Meanwhile, combine the mayonnaise, garlic, and mustard in a small bowl. Lightly stir in the basil and cheeses until just blended. Spoon equal amounts on each bread slice (about 1 slightly rounded teaspoon measure each piece), spread evenly over each slice. Return to oven for 3 minutes or until cheese has melted.

EXCHANGES / CHOICES	BASIC NUTRITIONAL VALUES			
1 Starch	**Calories**	115	**Potassium**	45 mg
1 Fat	Calories from Fat	35	**Total Carbohydrate**	16 g
	Total Fat	4.0 g	Dietary Fiber	1 g
	Saturated Fat	1.2 g	Sugars	2 g
	Trans Fat	0.0 g	**Protein**	5 g
	Cholesterol	5 mg	**Phosphorus**	110 mg
	Sodium	270 mg		

SERVES: 2
SERVING SIZE: 1 cup

Sneaky Strawberry Sipper

1 Combine all ingredients in blender.

2 Purée until smooth.

1 **cup** frozen unsweetened strawberries, thawed
$^1/_2$ **cup** frozen sliced carrots
1 (6-ounce) can pineapple juice

COOK'S TIP: You get 70% of your daily requirement of Vitamin A and 90% Vitamin C in every serving!

EXCHANGES / CHOICES
1 Fruit
1 Vegetable

BASIC NUTRITIONAL VALUES

Calories	80	**Potassium**	295 mg
Calories from Fat	0	**Total Carbohydrate**	20 g
Total Fat	0.0 g	Dietary Fiber	3 g
Saturated Fat	0.0 g	Sugars	13 g
Trans Fat	0.0 g	**Protein**	1 g
Cholesterol	0 mg	**Phosphorus**	25 mg
Sodium	25 mg		

Skillet Toasted Snackers

2 cups chex-style wheat or corn cereal
2 ounces rye melba rounds, broken into
  bite-size pieces
1/2 cup slivered almonds
1/3 cup hulled pumpkin seeds
1 tablespoon canola oil
1 tablespoon prepared mustard
1 tablespoon Worcestershire sauce
1 tablespoon smoked paprika
1/2 teaspoon salt

1 Heat a large nonstick skillet over medium-high heat. Add the cereal and melba pieces, almonds, and pumpkin seeds and cook 3 minutes or until beginning to turn golden brown, stirring frequently.

2 Whisk together the oil, mustard, and Worcestershire in a small bowl, drizzle over the cereal mixture, sprinkle evenly with the paprika and salt, and toss gently. Remove from heat and cool completely.

COOK'S TIP: To cool cereal mixture quickly, place on a sheet of foil in a single layer, let stand 10 minutes.

EXCHANGES / CHOICES
1 Starch
1 1/2 Fat

BASIC NUTRITIONAL VALUES

Calories	145	**Potassium**	165 mg
Calories from Fat	70	**Total Carbohydrate**	15 g
Total Fat	8.0 g	Dietary Fiber	3 g
Saturated Fat	0.9 g	Sugars	2 g
Trans Fat	0.0 g	**Protein**	5 g
Cholesterol	0 mg	**Phosphorus**	125 mg
Sodium	315 mg		

Garlic Bread Crisps

1 Preheat oven to 350°F. Arrange the bread slices in a single layer on a large baking sheet. Bake 3-4 minutes or until just beginning to brown on the bottom.

2 Combine the remaining ingredients, except the cheese, in a small bowl, brush the oil mixture evenly over all, and sprinkle with parmesan.

4 ounces whole-grain baguette bread, cut into 24 thin slices (about $^1/_8$-inch-thick slices)
2 tablespoons extra virgin olive oil
$^1/_2$ medium garlic clove, minced
$^1/_2$ **teaspoon** dried dill
$^1/_2$ **teaspoon** to **1 teaspoon** grated lemon zest
$^1/_8$ **teaspoon** dried pepper flakes (optional)
1 tablespoon grated Parmesan cheese

COOK'S TIP: This is a versatile and "make-ahead" recipe. May serve warm or at room temperature, as an appetizer or a side dish, and may be stored in an airtight container up to 3 days.

EXCHANGES / CHOICES	BASIC NUTRITIONAL VALUES			
$^1/_2$ Starch	**Calories**	90	**Potassium**	50 mg
1 Fat	Calories from Fat	45	**Total Carbohydrate**	8 g
	Total Fat	5.0 g	Dietary Fiber	1 g
	Saturated Fat	0.8 g	Sugars	1 g
	Trans Fat	0.0 g	**Protein**	3 g
	Cholesterol	0 mg	**Phosphorus**	45 mg
	Sodium	85 mg		

Potato Bites with Creamy Mustard Herb Dip

SERVES: 8

SERVING SIZE: $^1/_3$ cup potatoes and 1 tablespoon dip per serving

Dip

$^1/_4$ **cup** light mayonnaise
$^1/_4$ **cup** fat-free sour cream
1 **medium** garlic clove, minced
1 **teaspoon** dried oregano leaves
1 **teaspoon** Dijon mustard

Potatoes

1 **pound** red potatoes, cut in 1-inch
    chunks
2 **teaspoons** canola oil
$^1/_4$ **teaspoon** salt
$^1/_4$ **teaspoon** black pepper

1 Preheat oven to 425°F. Meanwhile, whisk together the dip ingredients and set aside.

2 Toss potatoes with oil on a foil-lined baking sheet, arrange in a single layer, sprinkle with salt and pepper, and bake 15 minutes or until tender when pierced with a fork. Serve with wooden toothpicks to pierce pieces.

EXCHANGES / CHOICES	BASIC NUTRITIONAL VALUES			
$^1/_2$ Starch	**Calories**	80	**Potassium**	270 mg
$^1/_2$ Carbohydrate	Calories from Fat	25	**Total Carbohydrate**	11 g
$^1/_2$ Fat	**Total Fat**	3.0 g	Dietary Fiber	1 g
	Saturated Fat	0.4 g	Sugars	2 g
	Trans Fat	0.0 g	**Protein**	1 g
	Cholesterol	0 mg	**Phosphorus**	45 mg
	Sodium	160 mg		

Cheese Stuffed Petite Peppers

SERVES: 4
SERVING SIZE: 3 pepper halves

1 Preheat broiler. Meanwhile, arrange pepper halves on a foil-lined baking sheet, coated with cooking spray. Sprinkle evenly with the salt, place 2 pieces of cheese in each pepper half, sprinkle with paprika, and coat with cooking spray.

2 Broil no closer than 5 inches away from heat source for 3 minutes or until cheese has melted and is beginning to slightly brown on top. Remove, sprinkle with cilantro, and let stand 5 minutes before serving.

6 petite peppers, halved lengthwise, seeds removed
1/8 **teaspoon** salt
2 **sticks** reduced-fat string cheese, halved lengthwise and each half cut into 6 pieces
1/4 **teaspoon** smoked paprika
1 **tablespoon** finely chopped fresh cilantro (optional)

COOK'S TIP: To prevent the peppers from "tilting" on baking sheet, you may want to slightly crumple a sheet of foil and line the baking sheet with the foil. Top with the pepper halves.

EXCHANGES / CHOICES
1/2 Fat

BASIC NUTRITIONAL VALUES

Calories	30	**Potassium**	50 mg
Calories from Fat	15	**Total Carbohydrate**	2 g
Total Fat	1.5 g	Dietary Fiber	0 g
Saturated Fat	0.8 g	Sugars	1 g
Trans Fat	0.0 g	**Protein**	3 g
Cholesterol	5 mg	**Phosphorus**	55 mg
Sodium	165 mg		

Avocado Cilantro Rounds

SERVES: 4
SERVING SIZE: ¹/₄ cup avocado mixture plus 6 cucumber slices

1 ripe medium avocado, diced
¹/₄ **cup** finely chopped fresh cilantro
2 **tablespoons** finely chopped red onion
1 **tablespoon** lime juice
¹/₄ **teaspoon** salt
1 large cucumber, cut into 24 slices

1 Combine all the avocado, cilantro, onion, juice, and salt in a small bowl, toss gently until well blended.

2 Spoon equal amounts (about 2 teaspoons) on each cucumber slice.

COOK'S TIP: For variation, use 6 medium plum tomatoes, cut into 4 rounds each.

EXCHANGES / CHOICES	BASIC NUTRITIONAL VALUES			
1 Vegetable	**Calories**	80	**Potassium**	360 mg
1 Fat	Calories from Fat	55	**Total Carbohydrate**	8 g
	Total Fat	6.0 g	Dietary Fiber	3 g
	Saturated Fat	0.8 g	Sugars	2 g
	Trans Fat	0.0 g	**Protein**	2 g
	Cholesterol	0 mg	**Phosphorus**	50 mg
	Sodium	150 mg		

Peach-Mango Wine Slush

SERVES: 13
SERVING SIZE: 3/4 cup per serving

1 Combine all the ingredients in a blender and purée until smooth. Pour into a gallon-size resealable plastic bag or other airtight container, cover, and freeze overnight. (Note: if using a resealable bag, place on a baking sheet on its side for support.)

2 When frozen, shave with fork or break up large pieces with a knife, reseal the baggie, and crush with your hands to create a "slush" effect. Store unused portion in freezer.

1 (15-ounce) can peach slices in own juice, undrained
1 (16-ounce) bag frozen mango chunks
2 cups frozen red raspberries
1 cup dry white wine
1/4 cup pourable sugar substitute

COOK'S TIP: May replace wine with 1 cup apple juice. If using juice, the frozen mixture will have to stand on kitchen counter 20 minutes to soften slightly and be shaved each time it's served. The wine mixture will retain a "shaved" texture when returned to the freezer because of the alcohol.

EXCHANGES / CHOICES
1 Fruit

BASIC NUTRITIONAL VALUES

Calories	70	Potassium	155 mg
Calories from Fat	0	Total Carbohydrate	14 g
Total Fat	0.0 g	Dietary Fiber	1 g
Saturated Fat	0.0 g	Sugars	13 g
Trans Fat	0.0 g	Protein	0 g
Cholesterol	0 mg	Phosphorus	20 mg
Sodium	0 mg		

SIDE SALADS

Tomato-Bread Salad

4 **ounces** whole or multigrain Italian
   bread, (preferably stale bread), cut
   into 1-inch cubes

2 medium tomatoes (8 ounces total),
   cut into 1-inch pieces

1 **cup** packed chopped kale

⅓ **cup** finely chopped red onion

1½ **ounces** reduced-fat feta, crumbled

1 **tablespoon** capers, drained

¼ **cup** chopped fresh basil

1 **tablespoon** extra virgin olive oil

1 **tablespoon** balsamic vinegar

1 medium garlic clove, minced

1 Place bread cubes on a baking sheet in a single layer.
   Turn on oven to 350°F (preheating is not needed).
   Bake 10 minutes or until firm. Cool 10 minutes.

2 Combine remaining ingredients in a bowl. Add the bread
   and toss. Let stand 5 minutes to absorb flavors and for
   bread to soften slightly.

COOK'S TIP: Serve immediately after the salad stands for 5 minutes for
peak flavor and texture.

EXCHANGES / CHOICES	BASIC NUTRITIONAL VALUES			
1 Starch	Calories	155	Potassium	345 mg
1 Vegetable	Calories from Fat	55	**Total Carbohydrate**	19 g
1 Fat	**Total Fat**	6.0 g	Dietary Fiber	4 g
	Saturated Fat	1.5 g	Sugars	6 g
	Trans Fat	0.0 g	**Protein**	8 g
	Cholesterol	5 mg	**Phosphorus**	140 mg
	Sodium	320 mg		

Marinated Veggie Salad

Serves: 4
Serving Size: 1 cup marinated vegetables and
3/4 cup greens per serving

1 Combine all ingredients, except spinach, in a shallow pan, such as a 13 × 9-inch glass baking dish. Cover and refrigerate 2 hours or overnight.

2 At time of serving, place equal amounts of the spinach on 4 salad plates. Spoon equal amounts of the salad on top of each.

1 (13.75-ounce) can quartered artichoke hearts, drained
4 ounces whole mushrooms, wiped clean with damp paper towels
1/3 cup diced red onion
1/2 medium cucumber, chopped
2 teaspoons dried dill
1/4 cup white balsamic vinegar
1 tablespoon extra virgin olive oil
1/4 teaspoon salt
2 cups packed spinach leaves or spring greens

Cook's Tip: For variation, use 4 bibb lettuce leaves instead of the spinach. They will act as "cups" to hold the marinated vegetables and their juices. It makes an impressive presentation . . . easy!

EXCHANGES / CHOICES	BASIC NUTRITIONAL VALUES			
3 Vegetable	**Calories**	110	**Potassium**	450 mg
1 Fat	Calories from Fat	35	**Total Carbohydrate**	16 g
	Total Fat	4.0 g	Dietary Fiber	4 g
	Saturated Fat	0.6 g	Sugars	6 g
	Trans Fat	0.0 g	**Protein**	4 g
	Cholesterol	0 mg	**Phosphorus**	95 mg
	Sodium	350 mg		

Fennel and Pear Salad

SERVES: 4
SERVING SIZE: 2 cups salad and 2 tablespoons dressing per serving

6 cups spring greens
1 cup thinly sliced fennel bulb, about 4 ounces
1 cup thinly sliced firm pear

Dressing

$1/4$ **cup** white balsamic vinegar
2 tablespoons canola oil
2 tablespoons strawberry fruit spread
$1/2$ **teaspoon** almond extract
$1/4$ **teaspoon** salt
$1/4$ **teaspoon** black pepper

1 Arrange equal amounts of the spring greens on 4 individual salad plates. Top with equal amounts of the fennel and pear slices.

2 Whisk together the salad dressing ingredients and spoon evenly over all.

EXCHANGES / CHOICES	BASIC NUTRITIONAL VALUES			
1 Fruit	Calories	140	Potassium	370 mg
1 Vegetable	Calories from Fat	65	**Total Carbohydrate**	19 g
1 1/2 Fat	**Total Fat**	7.0 g	Dietary Fiber	3 g
	Saturated Fat	0.5 g	Sugars	12 g
	Trans Fat	0.0 g	**Protein**	2 g
	Cholesterol	0 mg	**Phosphorus**	40 mg
	Sodium	185 mg		

Crisp Broccoli-Apple Salad

SERVES: 6
SERVING SIZE: $^2/_3$ cup

1 Combine all ingredients in a medium bowl.

2 Serve immediately or cover and refrigerate 1 hour to allow the curry to give the dish a refreshing yellow color.

2 cups small broccoli florets (about $^3/_4$-inch pieces)
$^1/_2$ **cup** diced tart apple, such as Granny Smith
1 medium celery stalk with leaves, diced
$^1/_4$ **cup** diced red onion
3 ounces ($^3/_4$ **cup**) chopped walnuts
$^1/_3$ **cup** reduced-sugar dried cranberries
$^1/_2$ **cup** nonfat vanilla yogurt
1 tablespoon lemon juice
1 teaspoon curry powder
$^1/_8$ **teaspoon** salt

EXCHANGES / CHOICES
$^1/_2$ Fruit
$^1/_2$ Carbohydrate
2 Fat

BASIC NUTRITIONAL VALUES

Calories	145	**Potassium**	225 mg
Calories from Fat	90	**Total Carbohydrate**	15 g
Total Fat	10.0 g	Dietary Fiber	4 g
Saturated Fat	1.0 g	Sugars	7 g
Trans Fat	0.0 g	**Protein**	4 g
Cholesterol	0 mg	**Phosphorus**	90 mg
Sodium	70 mg		

Heart of Palm and Avocado Salad

SERVES: 6
SERVING SIZE: $^3/_4$ cup

1 (14.1-ounce) can hearts of palm, drained and cut into $^1/_2$-inch slices
1 medium red bell pepper, coarsely chopped into $^3/_4$-inch cubes
$^1/_2$ medium English cucumber, quartered lengthwise and cut into $^3/_4$-inch chunks
2 ripe medium avocados, peeled, pitted, and chopped
$^1/_2$ **cup** diced red onion
1 to **2 teaspoons** sugar
$^1/_2$ **teaspoon** dried tarragon
2 tablespoons white balsamic vinegar
2 teaspoons canola oil
$^1/_4$ **teaspoon** black pepper
$^1/_4$ **teaspoon** salt

1   Combine all ingredients in a large bowl.

2   Cover and refrigerate 1 hour to allow flavors to absorb.

EXCHANGES / CHOICES	BASIC NUTRITIONAL VALUES			
$^1/_2$ Carbohydrate	**Calories**	140	**Potassium**	1020 mg
1 Vegetable	Calories from Fat	80	**Total Carbohydrate**	13 g
2 Fat	**Total Fat**	9.0 g	Dietary Fiber	5 g
	Saturated Fat	1.2 g	Sugars	6 g
	Trans Fat	0.0 g	**Protein**	3 g
	Cholesterol	0 mg	**Phosphorus**	95 mg
	Sodium	200 mg		

Rosemary Tomato Salad with Spinach

1 Combine all ingredients, except the cheese, in a medium bowl. Toss until well blended.

2 Sprinkle with the cheese.

10 ounces grape tomatoes, halved
2 cups (packed) baby spinach. coarsely chopped
16 pitted kalamata olives, coarsely chopped
¼ cup chopped fresh basil
2 teaspoons chopped fresh rosemary
1 tablespoon canola oil
1 tablespoon cider vinegar
½ medium garlic clove, minced
⅛ teaspoon salt
⅛ teaspoon dried pepper flakes
1 ounce thinly sliced reduced-fat Swiss cheese, cut into ½-inch pieces

EXCHANGES / CHOICES

1 Vegetable
1 ½ Fat

BASIC NUTRITIONAL VALUES

Calories	100	**Potassium**	275 mg
Calories from Fat	70	**Total Carbohydrate**	5 g
Total Fat	8.0 g	Dietary Fiber	2 g
Saturated Fat	1.2 g	Sugars	2 g
Trans Fat	0.0 g	**Protein**	4 g
Cholesterol	5 mg	**Phosphorus**	70 mg
Sodium	215 mg		

Corn and Black Bean Salsa Salad

SERVES: 6
SERVING SIZE: 3/4 cup

1 (14.5-ounce) can no-salt-added diced
   tomatoes, drained (see cook's tip)
1 (15-ounce) can no-salt-added black
   beans, rinsed and drained
1 cup diced red onion
1 cup frozen, thawed corn kernels
1/2 medium cucumber, peeled and
   chopped
1 jalapeño, minced
1/2 **cup** chopped fresh cilantro
1/2 **cup** fat-free Italian salad dressing
1/4 **cup** lime juice
1 teaspoon ground cumin

1   Combine all the ingredients. Serve immediately or cover
   and refrigerate up to 2 hours for peak flavors and texture.

COOK'S TIP: To make this a salsa, do not drain tomatoes.

EXCHANGES / CHOICES	BASIC NUTRITIONAL VALUES			
1 Starch	Calories	115	Potassium	440 mg
1 Vegetable	Calories from Fat	5	**Total Carbohydrate**	24 g
	Total Fat	0.5 g	Dietary Fiber	4 g
	Saturated Fat	0.2 g	Sugars	6 g
	Trans Fat	0.0 g	**Protein**	5 g
	Cholesterol	0 mg	**Phosphorus**	130 mg
	Sodium	240 mg		

Mexican Chop Salad

SERVES: 4
SERVING SIZE: 2 cups

1 Combine the romaine, tomato, poblano, cucumber, onion, cilantro, avocado, and cheese in a large bowl. Toss until well blended.

2 Combine the salad dressing, juice, and salt, pour over the lettuce mixture, and toss gently until well blended.

4 cups chopped romaine lettuce
1 cup diced tomato
1 medium poblano chili pepper, seeded and diced
1 cup chopped cucumber
1/3 cup diced red onion
1/4 cup chopped fresh cilantro
1 ripe avocado, peeled and chopped
3 tablespoons crumbled reduced-fat feta cheese
1/3 cup fat-free ranch-style dressing
2 tablespoons lime juice
1/8 teaspoon salt

EXCHANGES / CHOICES
1/2 Carbohydrate
2 Vegetable
1 Fat

BASIC NUTRITIONAL VALUES

Calories	130	**Potassium**	560 mg
Calories from Fat	65	**Total Carbohydrate**	17 g
Total Fat	7.0 g	Dietary Fiber	5 g
Saturated Fat	1.4 g	Sugars	6 g
Trans Fat	0.0 g	**Protein**	4 g
Cholesterol	5 mg	**Phosphorus**	110 mg
Sodium	385 mg		

Greek Greens

Salad

$1/2$ (10-ounce) bag torn romaine lettuce
12 pitted kalamata olives, coarsely
    chopped
1 cup sliced cucumber
1 cup chopped tomato
$1/3$ **cup** thinly sliced red onion
1 ounce reduced-fat feta cheese,
    crumbled

Dressing

$1\,1/2$ **tablespoons** cider vinegar
2 tablespoons dry white wine
2 tablespoons canola oil
1 medium garlic clove, minced
$1\,1/2$ **teaspoons** dried oregano leaves
$1/8$ **teaspoon** dried pepper flakes
$1/4$ **teaspoon** salt

1   Combine the salad ingredients in a large bowl.

2   Whisk together the dressing ingredients in a small
bowl, pour over the salad ingredients, and toss until well
blended.

**EXCHANGES /
CHOICES**

1 Vegetable
2 Fat

BASIC NUTRITIONAL VALUES

Calories	125	**Potassium**	270 mg
Calories from Fat	90	**Total Carbohydrate**	6 g
Total Fat	10.0 g	Dietary Fiber	2 g
Saturated Fat	1.3 g	Sugars	3 g
Trans Fat	0.0 g	**Protein**	3 g
Cholesterol	5 mg	**Phosphorus**	55 mg
Sodium	330 mg		

Creamy Sweet Pea Coleslaw

SERVES: 4
SERVING SIZE: ³/₄ cup

1 Combine all ingredients in a large bowl. Stir until well blended.

2 Cover and refrigerate 1 hour before serving.

¹/₂ (14-ounce) bag coleslaw
1 cup frozen green peas, thawed
¹/₄ **cup** plain nonfat Greek yogurt
3 tablespoons light mayonnaise
1 tablespoon plus 1 teaspoon sugar
2 teaspoons cider vinegar
¹/₄ **teaspoon** salt
¹/₈ **teaspoon** black pepper

EXCHANGES / CHOICES

1 Carbohydrate
¹/₂ Fat

BASIC NUTRITIONAL VALUES

Calories	95	**Potassium**	200 mg
Calories from Fat	25	**Total Carbohydrate**	14 g
Total Fat	3.0 g	Dietary Fiber	3 g
Saturated Fat	0.4 g	Sugars	8 g
Trans Fat	0.0 g	**Protein**	3 g
Cholesterol	0 mg	**Phosphorus**	60 mg
Sodium	290 mg		

Raspberry-Lime Watermelon

4 **cups** watermelon cubes
2 **tablespoons** raspberry fruit spread
1½ **tablespoons** lime juice
1½ **tablespoons** finely chopped fresh
    mint or cilantro (optional)

1 Place watermelon in a shallow serving bowl.

2 Place fruit spread and juice in a small microwave-safe bowl and microwave on high setting for 30 seconds or until fruit spread has melted. Whisk together until smooth. Spoon evenly over the watermelon. Sprinkle with mint or cilantro, if desired.

COOK'S TIP: This may be served as a snack as well.

EXCHANGES / CHOICES

1 Fruit

BASIC NUTRITIONAL VALUES

Calories	65	**Potassium**	180 mg
Calories from Fat	0	**Total Carbohydrate**	17 g
Total Fat	0.0 g	Dietary Fiber	1 g
Saturated Fat	0.0 g	Sugars	14 g
Trans Fat	0.0 g	**Protein**	1 g
Cholesterol	0 mg	**Phosphorus**	20 mg
Sodium	0 mg		

SERVES: 4
SERVING SIZE: ³/₄ cup

Kiwi, Blueberry, and Pear Salad

1   Place equal amounts of the pear on 4 salad plates. Sprinkle evenly with the mint and top with the kiwi and blueberries.

2   Combine the juice, sugar, and ginger in a small jar, secure with lid, and shake vigorously until well blended. Spoon evenly over all.

1 firm medium pear, halved, cored, and sliced
¹/₄ **cup** chopped fresh mint
1 ripe medium kiwi, peeled and sliced
¹/₂ **cup** blueberries
3 **tablespoons** fresh lemon juice
1 **tablespoon** sugar
1 **teaspoon** grated ginger

EXCHANGES / CHOICES

1 Fruit

BASIC NUTRITIONAL VALUES

Calories	65	**Potassium**	150 mg
Calories from Fat	0	**Total Carbohydrate**	16 g
Total Fat	0.0 g	Dietary Fiber	3 g
Saturated Fat	0.0 g	Sugars	11 g
Trans Fat	0.0 g	**Protein**	1 g
Cholesterol	0 mg	**Phosphorus**	15 mg
Sodium	0 mg		

Sweet Cream Tropical Salad with Coconut

Serves: 4
Serving Size: ³/₄ cup

¹/₂ **cup** fat-free sour cream
1 **tablespoon** sugar substitute
¹/₂ **teaspoon** vanilla
1 **cup** fresh or frozen, thawed chopped
    mango
1 **cup** fresh pineapple chunks
1 **cup** strawberries, quartered
3 **tablespoons** flaked sweetened coconut

1   Stir together the sour cream, sugar substitute, and vanilla
    in a large bowl. Gently stir in remaining ingredients.

2   Let stand 10 minutes to allow flavors to blend.

EXCHANGES / CHOICES	BASIC NUTRITIONAL VALUES			
1 Fruit	**Calories**	110	**Potassium**	235 mg
¹/₂ Carbohydrate	Calories from Fat	20	**Total Carbohydrate**	23 g
¹/₂ Fat	**Total Fat**	2.0 g	Dietary Fiber	2 g
	Saturated Fat	1.5 g	Sugars	16 g
	Trans Fat	0.0 g	**Protein**	2 g
	Cholesterol	5 mg	**Phosphorus**	55 mg
	Sodium	45 mg		

SIDES
(VEGETABLES AND FRUITS AND GRAINS)

Lemon-Walnut Minted Rice

$^3/_4$ **cup** water
$^1/_2$ **cup** fast-cooking brown rice
1 ounce chopped walnuts
2 teaspoons grated lemon zest
$^1/_4$ **cup** chopped fresh mint
$^1/_4$ **teaspoon** salt
2 teaspoons canola oil

1 Bring water to a boil in a medium saucepan. Stir in the rice, reduce heat to medium low, cover, and cook 10 minutes or until water is absorbed. Remove from heat.

2 Stir in the remaining ingredients.

EXCHANGES / CHOICES

1 Starch
1 Fat

BASIC NUTRITIONAL VALUES

Calories	130	**Potassium**	80 mg
Calories from Fat	65	**Total Carbohydrate**	14 g
Total Fat	7.0 g	Dietary Fiber	2 g
Saturated Fat	0.6 g	Sugars	0 g
Trans Fat	0.0 g	**Protein**	3 g
Cholesterol	0 mg	**Phosphorus**	75 mg
Sodium	155 mg		

Toasted Almond, Roasted Asparagus

SERVES: 4
SERVING SIZE: 6 asparagus spears and 2 tablespoons almonds

1 Preheat oven to 425°F. Coat a baking sheet with cooking spray, arrange the asparagus in a single layer on baking sheet, coat the asparagus with cooking spray. Roast 5 minutes or until just beginning to brown.

2 Turn asparagus, sprinkle the almonds around asparagus, sprinkle with the salt and pepper, and bake 4–5 minutes or until almonds are beginning to lightly brown. Sprinkle with the soy sauce.

Cooking spray
1 pound asparagus spears, ends trimmed
2 ounces sliced almonds
$1/8$ teaspoon salt
$1/8$ teaspoon black pepper
2 teaspoons light soy sauce

EXCHANGES / CHOICES	BASIC NUTRITIONAL VALUES			
$1/2$ Carbohydrate	**Calories**	100	**Potassium**	230 mg
$1 1/2$ Fat	Calories from Fat	70	**Total Carbohydrate**	6 g
	Total Fat	8.0 g	Dietary Fiber	3 g
	Saturated Fat	0.6 g	Sugars	1 g
	Trans Fat	0.0 g	**Protein**	5 g
	Cholesterol	0 mg	**Phosphorus**	100 mg
	Sodium	170 mg		

Lemon-Dilled Artichokes Halves

10 **cups** water

1 **tablespoon** cider vinegar

2 medium whole artichokes, about
8 ounces each, trimmed and halved
lengthwise

Sauce

1/4 **cup** lower-fat (<50% vegetable oil)
margarine-type spread, softened

2 **teaspoons** grated lemon zest

2 **teaspoons** chopped fresh dill

1/4 **teaspoon** salt

1 medium lemon, quartered

1 In a large stock pot, bring the water and vinegar to a boil over high heat. Place the artichokes in the boiling water. Return to a boil. Reduce the heat to medium, cover, and cook for 30 minutes, or until leaves can easily be pulled off. Drain on paper towels, cut side down.

2 Meanwhile, in a small bowl, whisk together the sauce ingredients, except the lemon wedges. Arrange the artichokes, cut side up, on a large plate. Gently scrape out and discard the choke (or inedible prickly center). Brush or spoon the sauce evenly over the artichokes. Serve with the lemon wedges.

COOK'S TIP: To cut the artichokes in half easily, it's best to use a serrated knife. (They cook in a fraction of the time it takes to cook whole artichokes!)

EXCHANGES / CHOICES	BASIC NUTRITIONAL VALUES			
1 Vegetable	Calories	75	Potassium	145 mg
1 Fat	Calories from Fat	45	Total Carbohydrate	6 g
	Total Fat	5.0 g	Dietary Fiber	4 g
	Saturated Fat	1.2 g	Sugars	1 g
	Trans Fat	0.0 g	Protein	1 g
	Cholesterol	0 mg	Phosphorus	35 mg
	Sodium	265 mg		

Roasted Green Beans, Parsnips, and Garlic

SERVES: 4
SERVING SIZE: ³/₄ cup

1 Preheat oven 425°F. Place the beans, parsnips, and garlic on a foil-lined baking sheet. Drizzle with the oil, lightly toss to coat, and arrange in a single layer.

2 Roast for 15 minutes or until beginning to brown on edges. Sprinkle evenly with tarragon and salt. Note: If time allows, seal vegetables in the foil they were cooked on and let stand 5 minutes to absorb flavors and for all the natural juices to develop.

8 ounces green beans, cut into 2-inch pieces
8 ounces parsnips, peeled, quartered lengthwise, and cut into 2-inch pieces
8 garlic cloves, peeled only
1 ¹/₂ tablespoons extra virgin olive oil
¹/₂ teaspoon dried tarragon leaves
¹/₂ teaspoon salt

EXCHANGES / CHOICES

¹/₂ Starch
1 Vegetable
1 Fat

BASIC NUTRITIONAL VALUES

Calories	105	**Potassium**	275 mg
Calories from Fat	45	**Total Carbohydrate**	14 g
Total Fat	5.0 g	Dietary Fiber	3 g
Saturated Fat	0.8 g	Sugars	3 g
Trans Fat	0.0 g	**Protein**	2 g
Cholesterol	0 mg	**Phosphorus**	55 mg
Sodium	295 mg		

Sweet Orange-Scented Carrots

SERVES: 4
SERVING SIZE: $^3/_4$ cup

3 cups water
1 pound carrots, peeled and sliced
1 1/2 teaspoons grated orange zest
2 tablespoons lower-fat (<50% vegetable oil) margarine-type spread
2 tablespoons packed dark brown sugar
1 teaspoon Dijon mustard
1/4 teaspoon salt

1 Add water to a large saucepan. Place collapsible steamer basket in saucepan. Arrange carrots in basket. Cover and bring to a boil over high heat. Cook 8 minutes or until carrots are tender crisp.

2 Remove carrots from steamer basket, place in medium bowl, and toss with remaining ingredients.

EXCHANGES / CHOICES

1/2 Carbohydrate
2 Vegetable
1/2 Fat

BASIC NUTRITIONAL VALUES

Calories	90	**Potassium**	335 mg
Calories from Fat	25	**Total Carbohydrate**	17 g
Total Fat	3.0 g	Dietary Fiber	3 g
Saturated Fat	0.6 g	Sugars	12 g
Trans Fat	0.0 g	**Protein**	1 g
Cholesterol	0 mg	**Phosphorus**	40 mg
Sodium	290 mg		

Skillet Tossed Garlic Brussels Sprouts

1 Add water to a large nonstick skillet. Bring to a boil over medium-high heat, add the Brussels sprouts, return to a boil, reduce heat to medium-low, cover, and cook 10–12 minutes or until sprouts are tender crisp. Drain well, discarding liquid.

2 Return Brussels sprouts to the skillet with remaining ingredients. Cook over medium-high heat until liquid is absorbed, about 3-4 minutes, stirring frequently.

2 cups water

12 ounces fresh or frozen Brussels sprouts (ends trimmed, if fresh)

3 tablespoons lower-fat (<50% vegetable oil) margarine-type spread

1–2 medium garlic cloves, minced

1 teaspoon Worcestershire sauce

$^1/_4$ teaspoon salt

$^1/_8$ teaspoon black pepper

EXCHANGES / CHOICES	BASIC NUTRITIONAL VALUES			
1 Vegetable	**Calories**	65	**Potassium**	285 mg
1 Fat	Calories from Fat	35	**Total Carbohydrate**	7 g
	Total Fat	4.0 g	Dietary Fiber	2 g
	Saturated Fat	0.9 g	Sugars	2 g
	Trans Fat	0.0 g	**Protein**	2 g
	Cholesterol	0 mg	**Phosphorus**	50 mg
	Sodium	240 mg		

Roasted Root Veggies with Blue Cheese

SERVES: 4
SERVING SIZE: $^3/_4$ cup

12 ounces red potatoes, quartered
1 cup coarsely chopped onion
3 medium carrots, cut into 1-inch
    chunks
1 tablespoon canola oil
$^1/_4$ **teaspoon** dried oregano
$^1/_4$ **teaspoon** salt
$^1/_8$ **teaspoon** dried pepper flakes
1 ounce reduced-fat blue cheese,
    crumbled

1 Preheat oven to 425°F. Meanwhile, combine all
   ingredients, except the cheese, on a foil-lined baking
   sheet. Toss until well blended and arrange in a single
   layer.

2 Roast 24 minutes or until carrots are just tender. Remove
   from oven and sprinkle evenly with the cheese.

COOK'S TIP: If time allows, fold the ends up and gently wrap the
vegetables after topping with the cheese. Let stand 5 minutes to allow
the flavors to blend and the natural juices to be released, providing a
moister texture to the dish.

EXCHANGES / CHOICES
1 Starch
1 Vegetable
1 Fat

BASIC NUTRITIONAL VALUES

Calories	150	**Potassium**	600 mg
Calories from Fat	45	**Total Carbohydrate**	22 g
Total Fat	5.0 g	Dietary Fiber	3 g
Saturated Fat	1.2 g	Sugars	5 g
Trans Fat	0.0 g	**Protein**	4 g
Cholesterol	5 mg	**Phosphorus**	105 mg
Sodium	285 mg		

Dill Asparagus Pasta

Serves: 4
Serving Size: ³/₄ cup

3 **ounces** multi-grain rotini pasta
6 **ounces** asparagus, cut in 2-inch pieces
1 **tablespoon** extra virgin olive oil
1 **medium** garlic clove, minced
1 **tablespoon** grated lemon zest
2 **teaspoons** dried dill weed
¹/₄ **teaspoon** salt
¹/₈ **teaspoon** black pepper

1 Cook pasta according to package directions, adding the asparagus to the pasta the last 2 minutes of cooking time. Drain well.

2 Combine the remaining ingredients in a medium bowl and stir in the pasta mixture until well blended.

Cook's Tip: To serve as a main salad, quickly cool the pasta and asparagus in a colander under cold water, drain well before adding pasta to the remaining ingredients, then stir in a 15-ounce can navy beans, rinsed and drained, or 1 ½ cups cooked diced chicken. Serve with lemon wedges for an extra boost of citrus!

EXCHANGES / CHOICES	BASIC NUTRITIONAL VALUES			
1 Starch	**Calories**	120	**Potassium**	155 mg
1 Fat	Calories from Fat	35	**Total Carbohydrate**	17 g
	Total Fat	4.0 g	Dietary Fiber	3 g
	Saturated Fat	0.6 g	Sugars	2 g
	Trans Fat	0.0 g	**Protein**	5 g
	Cholesterol	0 mg	**Phosphorus**	80 mg
	Sodium	155 mg		

Smoky Poblano Rice

1 tablespoon extra virgin olive oil, divided use
2 medium poblano chili peppers, seeded and diced
1 cup diced onion
1 ¹/₃ cups water
²/₃ cup instant brown rice
1 teaspoon smoked paprika
¹/₄ cup chopped fresh cilantro
¹/₂ teaspoon salt
1 medium lime, quartered

1 Heat 1 teaspoon of the oil in a large nonstick skillet over medium-high heat, add the chilies and onions, and cook 4 minutes or until onions are soft. Stir in the water, rice, and paprika, bring to a boil over medium-high heat, reduce heat to medium-low, cover, and cook 12 minutes or until water is absorbed.

2 Remove from heat, stir in the cilantro and salt. Serve with lime wedges.

EXCHANGES / CHOICES

1 ¹/₂ Starch
1 Vegetable
¹/₂ Fat

BASIC NUTRITIONAL VALUES

Calories	175	**Potassium**	265 mg
Calories from Fat	40	**Total Carbohydrate**	32 g
Total Fat	4.5 g	Dietary Fiber	3 g
Saturated Fat	0.6 g	Sugars	4 g
Trans Fat	0.0 g	**Protein**	4 g
Cholesterol	0 mg	**Phosphorus**	135 mg
Sodium	315 mg		

Zucchini-Red Pepper Corn

SERVES: 4
SERVING SIZE: $^3/_4$ cup

1 Heat 1 teaspoon of the oil in a large nonstick skillet over medium-high heat, add the onions, zucchini, and peppers and cook 8 minutes or until just browning on the edges.

2 Stir in remaining ingredients, cook 1 minute to heat through.

1 **tablespoon** extra virgin olive oil, divided use
$^1/_2$ **cup** diced onions
1 medium zucchini
1 **cup** diced red bell pepper
1 $^1/_2$ **cups** frozen corn, thawed
2 **tablespoons** finely chopped fresh parsley
$^1/_2$ **teaspoon** salt
$^1/_4$ **teaspoon** black pepper

EXCHANGES / CHOICES

1 Starch
1 Vegetable
$^1/_2$ Fat

BASIC NUTRITIONAL VALUES

Calories	120	**Potassium**	430 mg
Calories from Fat	35	**Total Carbohydrate**	21 g
Total Fat	4.0 g	Dietary Fiber	3 g
Saturated Fat	0.6 g	Sugars	6 g
Trans Fat	0.0 g	**Protein**	3 g
Cholesterol	0 mg	**Phosphorus**	90 mg
Sodium	300 mg		

Vanilla Honey Sweet Potatoes

Serves: 4
Serving Size: 1 potato half and 1 tablespoon honey mixture per serving

2 (8-ounce) sweet potatoes, pierced in several areas with a fork
3 tablespoons lower-fat (<50% vegetable oil) margarine-type spread
1 tablespoon honey
$^1/_2$ teaspoon vanilla
Dash of ground nutmeg
$^1/_8$ teaspoon salt

1 Wrap each potato in a paper towel and microwave on high setting for 10 minutes or until tender when pierced with a fork.

2 Combine the remaining ingredients in a small bowl. Cut potatoes in half lengthwise, fluff with a fork, and spoon equal amounts of the honey mixture on each.

EXCHANGES / CHOICES	BASIC NUTRITIONAL VALUES			
1 Starch	**Calories**	125	**Potassium**	395 mg
$^1/_2$ Carbohydrate	Calories from Fat	35	**Total Carbohydrate**	21 g
$^1/_2$ Fat	**Total Fat**	4.0 g	Dietary Fiber	3 g
	Saturated Fat	0.8 g	Sugars	10 g
	Trans Fat	0.0 g	**Protein**	2 g
	Cholesterol	0 mg	**Phosphorus**	45 mg
	Sodium	165 mg		

Coconut Almond Bulgur

1 Heat a medium saucepan over medium-high heat. Add the almonds and cook 2–3 minutes or until golden, stirring frequently. Remove from saucepan and set aside on separate plate.

2 Bring water, bulgur, and raisins to a boil in the saucepan over high heat, reduce heat to medium low, cover, and cook 12 minutes or until tender. Stir in almonds and remaining ingredients.

2 ounces slivered almonds
1 cup water
1/3 cup dry bulgur
2 tablespoons raisins
3 tablespoons flaked sweetened coconut
1/4 teaspoon ground cumin
Dash of cayenne (optional)
1/4 teaspoon salt

EXCHANGES / CHOICES

1 Carbohydrate
2 Fat

BASIC NUTRITIONAL VALUES

Calories	160	**Potassium**	200 mg
Calories from Fat	80	**Total Carbohydrate**	18 g
Total Fat	9.0 g	Dietary Fiber	4 g
Saturated Fat	1.5 g	Sugars	5 g
Trans Fat	0.0 g	**Protein**	5 g
Cholesterol	0 mg	**Phosphorus**	115 mg
Sodium	160 mg		

Veggie-Loaded Sweet Corn Muffins

SERVES: 8
SERVING SIZE: 1 muffin

1 (8.5-ounce) corn muffin mix, such as Jiffy
1/3 cup fat-free milk
1 large egg
1/3 cup finely chopped onions
1/2 cup frozen corn
1 medium poblano chili pepper, seeded and finely chopped
1 tablespoon extra virgin olive oil

1 Preheat oven to 400°F. Meanwhile, stir together the muffin mix, milk, and egg in a medium bowl. Spoon equal amounts into each of 8 nonstick muffin tins coated with cooking spray. Top with equal amounts of the remaining ingredients, except the oil. Drizzle oil evenly over all.

2 Bake 15–20 minutes or until wooden pick inserted comes out clean. Let stand 5 minutes before removing from pan. Cool completely on wire rack.

COOK'S TIP: Store leftovers in an airtight container up to 24 hours or freeze up to 2 weeks.

EXCHANGES / CHOICES
1 1/2 Starch
1/2 Fat

BASIC NUTRITIONAL VALUES

Calories	125	**Potassium**	115 mg
Calories from Fat	40	**Total Carbohydrate**	25 g
Total Fat	4.5 g	Dietary Fiber	1 g
Saturated Fat	1.6 g	Sugars	8 g
Trans Fat	0.0 g	**Protein**	3 g
Cholesterol	25 mg	**Phosphorus**	185 mg
Sodium	255 mg		

Double Onion Potatoes

Serves: 4
Serving Size: 1 cup

1 Bring water to boil over high heat in a large saucepan. Add potatoes and yellow onion, return to boil, reduce heat, cover, and boil for 6–8 minutes or until potatoes are tender; drain.

2 Return potatoes to pan (removed from heat), toss with remaining ingredients until margarine is melted.

4 cups water
1 pound red potatoes, chopped
1 cup diced yellow onion
1/3 cup chopped green onions
3 tablespoons lower-fat (<50% vegetable oil) margarine-type spread
1/2 teaspoon salt
1/4 teaspoon black pepper
1/8 teaspoon garlic powder

EXCHANGES / CHOICES

1 1/2 Starch
1 Vegetable
1/2 Fat

BASIC NUTRITIONAL VALUES

Calories	150	**Potassium**	505 mg
Calories from Fat	35	**Total Carbohydrate**	26 g
Total Fat	4.0 g	Dietary Fiber	3 g
Saturated Fat	0.9 g	Sugars	3 g
Trans Fat	0.0 g	**Protein**	3 g
Cholesterol	0 mg	**Phosphorus**	65 mg
Sodium	365 mg		

Sweet Potato Fries with Smoky Dipping Sauce

SERVES: 4
SERVING SIZE: $^3/_4$ cup potatoes and
2 tablespoons sauce per serving

Sauce

$^1/_4$ **cup** nonfat plain Greek yogurt
$^1/_4$ **cup** light mayonnaise
1 teaspoon ketchup
$^1/_4$ **teaspoon** smoked paprika
$^1/_8$ **teaspoon** salt

Potatoes

1 pound sweet potatoes, peeled, and cut
into $^1/_2$-inch thick rounds, and then
each round cut into $^1/_2$-inch thick
strips (resembling short thick-cut
French fries)
1 tablespoon canola oil
$^1/_4$ **teaspoon** salt
$^1/_4$ **teaspoon** black pepper

1 Preheat oven to 425°F. Meanwhile, whisk together the
sauce ingredients and set aside.

2 Toss potatoes with oil on a foil-lined baking sheet,
arrange in a single layer, sprinkle with salt and pepper and
bake 15 minutes or until tender when pierced with a fork.

EXCHANGES / CHOICES
1 Starch
1 $^1/_2$ Fat

BASIC NUTRITIONAL VALUES

Calories	145	**Potassium**	370 mg
Calories from Fat	65	**Total Carbohydrate**	17 g
Total Fat	7.0 g	Dietary Fiber	2 g
Saturated Fat	0.8 g	Sugars	6 g
Trans Fat	0.0 g	**Protein**	3 g
Cholesterol	5 mg	**Phosphorus**	65 mg
Sodium	380 mg		

ENTREES

Sweet Spiced Chili Bowls

Serves: 4
Serving Size: 1½ cups

1 **pound** extra-lean (90% lean) ground beef
3 **medium** poblano chilies, seeded and chopped
1 **cup** diced onion
1 (15.5-ounce) **can** no-salt-added dark kidney beans, rinsed and drained
1 (14.5-ounce) **can** no-salt-added stewed tomatoes
12 **ounces** light lager beer
⅓ **cup** ketchup
1 **tablespoon** smoked paprika
2 **teaspoons** ground cumin
½ **teaspoon** ground cinnamon
¼ **teaspoon** salt
½ **cup** finely chopped green onion

1 Heat a Dutch oven over medium-high heat. Cook the beef 3 minutes or until beginning to brown, stirring frequently. Drain any fat from meat. Stir in the remaining ingredients, except the green onions. Bring to a boil, reduce heat to medium-low, cover, and simmer 50–55 minutes or until thickened.

2 Serve sprinkle evenly with green onions.

Cook's Tip: Flavors improve overnight so this recipe is great made ahead of time.

EXCHANGES / CHOICES

1 Starch
½ Carbohydrate
3 Vegetable
3 Protein, lean
1 Fat

BASIC NUTRITIONAL VALUES

Calories	385	**Potassium**	1250 mg
Calories from Fat	90	**Total Carbohydrate**	40 g
Total Fat	10.0 g	Dietary Fiber	9 g
Saturated Fat	3.8 g	Sugars	16 g
Trans Fat	0.6 g	**Protein**	31 g
Cholesterol	70 mg	**Phosphorus**	375 mg
Sodium	485 mg		

Ground Beef and Noodle Skillet Casserole

1 Heat a large nonstick skillet over medium-high heat. Brown the beef for about 3 minutes, stirring frequently. Drain any fat from beef.

2 Stir in the remaining ingredients. Bring to a boil, reduce heat, cover, and cook over medium heat for 15 minutes or until noodles are cooked.

1 pound extra-lean (90% lean) ground beef
4 ounces multigrain or whole-grain rotini
1 (14.5-ounce) can no-salt-added stewed tomatoes
1 $1/2$ cups diced green bell pepper
4 ounces sliced mushrooms
$1/4$ cup ketchup
1 tablespoon Worcestershire sauce
1 tablespoon balsamic vinegar
$1/2$ cup water
$1/4$ teaspoon salt

COOK'S TIP: This is a great "throw and go" recipe ... and kids love it!

EXCHANGES / CHOICES
1 $1/2$ Starch
2 Vegetable
3 Protein, lean
1 Fat

BASIC NUTRITIONAL VALUES

Calories	345	**Potassium**	915 mg
Calories from Fat	90	**Total Carbohydrate**	36 g
Total Fat	10.0 g	Dietary Fiber	6 g
Saturated Fat	3.8 g	Sugars	12 g
Trans Fat	0.6 g	**Protein**	29 g
Cholesterol	70 mg	**Phosphorus**	330 mg
Sodium	470 mg		

Pot Roast with Burgundy

1 ½ **pounds** carrots, scrubbed and cut into thirds

12 **ounces** onions, cut into ¹⁄₂-inch wedges

1 (14.5-ounce) can no-salt-added stewed tomatoes, drained

2 ¹⁄₂ **pounds** trimmed lean boneless chuck roast

1 **cup** dry red wine

¹⁄₄ **cup** ketchup

1 ¹⁄₂ **tablespoons** Worcestershire sauce

1 ¹⁄₂ **tablespoons** balsamic vinegar

1 **tablespoon** sodium-free beef bouillon

1 **teaspoon** dried thyme leaves

2 medium dried bay leaves

1 **teaspoon** salt

¹⁄₂ **teaspoon** black pepper

1. Place all the ingredients in a 3¹⁄₂ to 4-quart slow cooker in the order above.

2. Cover and cook on high for 5¹⁄₂ to 6 hours. Remove bay leaves before serving.

COOK'S TIP: If desired, may bake in a roasting pan, covered, in a 325°F preheated oven for 5 hours or until very tender.

EXCHANGES / CHOICES

3 Vegetable
3 Protein, lean

BASIC NUTRITIONAL VALUES

Calories	210	**Potassium**	800 mg
Calories from Fat	35	**Total Carbohydrate**	17 g
Total Fat	4.0 g	Dietary Fiber	3 g
Saturated Fat	1.3 g	Sugars	10 g
Trans Fat	0.0 g	**Protein**	27 g
Cholesterol	45 mg	**Phosphorus**	205 mg
Sodium	505 mg		

Spiced Ground Beef and Almond and Raisins

Serves: 4
Serving Size: 1 cup beef mixture and 2 tablespoons yogurt

1 Heat a large nonstick skillet over medium-high heat. Brown the beef. Drain of any fat. Stir in the onions, bell pepper, eggplant, tomatoes, raisins, allspice, and cumin. Bring to a boil, reduce heat to medium-low, cover, and cook 30 minutes or until onions are very tender. Remove from heat.

2 Stir in the almonds, salt, and all but 2 tablespoons mint. Serve in shallow bowls to hold juices in and top with yogurt and remaining mint.

10 ounces extra-lean (90% lean) ground beef
1 cup diced yellow onion
1 medium red bell pepper, coarsely chopped (³/₄-inch pieces)
8 ounces eggplant, cut into ¹/₂-inch cubes
1 (14.5-ounce) can no-salt-added stewed tomatoes
¹/₄ cup dark raisins
1¹/₂ teaspoons ground allspice
1 teaspoon ground cumin
1 ounce slivered almonds, preferably toasted
¹/₂ teaspoon salt
1 cup chopped fresh mint, divided use
¹/₂ cup nonfat plain Greek yogurt

EXCHANGES / CHOICES

¹/₂ Fruit
4 Vegetable
2 Protein, lean
1¹/₂ Fat

BASIC NUTRITIONAL VALUES

Calories	280	**Potassium**	895 mg
Calories from Fat	90	**Total Carbohydrate**	30 g
Total Fat	10.0 g	Dietary Fiber	7 g
Saturated Fat	2.7 g	Sugars	18 g
Trans Fat	04 g	**Protein**	21 g
Cholesterol	45 mg	**Phosphorus**	265 mg
Sodium	395 mg		

Caldio-Style Stew

2 cans (14.5-ounce each) no-salt-added stewed tomatoes

1½ **pounds** new potatoes, halved lengthwise

2 medium onions (8 ounces total), cut into ½-inch wedges

2 **cans** (4.5 ounces each) chopped green chilies

1½ **pounds** trimmed extra-lean boneless chuck roast, cut into 1½-inch cubes

1 **teaspoon** Worcestershire sauce

1 **tablespoon** sodium-free beef bouillon granules

1 **tablespoon** smoked paprika

2 **teaspoons** garlic powder

1½ **teaspoons** ground cumin

¾ **teaspoon** salt

1 Drain 1 can of tomatoes and discard liquid. Place the drained tomatoes in bottom of a 3½ to 4-quart slow cooker with the potatoes, onion, chilies, and the remaining can of tomatoes and its liquid. Top with the chuck and sprinkle the remaining ingredients evenly over all.

2 Cover and cook on high for 5 to 5½ hours or until beef is fork tender.

COOK'S TIP: Have the butcher trim and cut the chuck. You may want to call ahead. Be sure to tell him that the weight you want is the weight AFTER it is trimmed of fat.

EXCHANGES / CHOICES

1½ Starch
3 Vegetable
3 Protein, lean

BASIC NUTRITIONAL VALUES

Calories	320	**Potassium**	1440 mg
Calories from Fat	70	**Total Carbohydrate**	38 g
Total Fat	8.0 g	Dietary Fiber	5 g
Saturated Fat	3.0 g	Sugars	10 g
Trans Fat	0.3 g	**Protein**	28 g
Cholesterol	80 mg	**Phosphorus**	325 mg
Sodium	605 mg		

Marinated Sweet Soy Flank

Serves: 6
Serving Size: 3 ounces cooked beef

1 Combine all ingredients, except green onion, in a gallon-size plastic bag, seal tightly and toss back and forth until well blended. Refrigerate 8 hours or up to 48 hours.

2 Heat grill pan over medium-high heat. Coat grill pan with cooking spray. Remove beef from marinade, discarding marinade. Pat dry beef with paper towels. Cook 4 minutes each side. (Note: do not cook any longer or it will become tough.) Place meat on cutting board and let stand 10 minutes before thinly slicing diagonally against the grain. Sprinkle with green onion, if desired.

$^1/_4$ **cup** light soy sauce
2 tablespoons ketchup
1 tablespoon balsamic vinegar
$^1/_2$ **teaspoon** garlic powder
$^1/_2$ **teaspoon** onion powder
$^1/_4$ **teaspoon** dried pepper flakes
1 $^1/_2$ pounds flank steak
2 tablespoons finely chopped green onion (optional)

Cook's Tip: If time allows, remove beef from refrigerator before cooking and let stand 15–20 minutes for more even cooking.

EXCHANGES / CHOICES
3 Protein, lean

BASIC NUTRITIONAL VALUES

Calories	155	**Potassium**	300 mg
Calories from Fat	55	**Total Carbohydrate**	1 g
Total Fat	6.0 g	Dietary Fiber	0 g
Saturated Fat	2.5 g	Sugars	1 g
Trans Fat	0.0 g	**Protein**	23 g
Cholesterol	60 mg	**Phosphorus**	180 mg
Sodium	230 mg		

Eye of Round Roast with Garlic Onions

SERVES: 8
SERVING SIZE: 3 ounces cooked beef and 2 tablespoons onion mixture

1 tablespoon instant coffee granules
1 tablespoon chili powder
1 teaspoon salt
1/2 teaspoon black pepper
1 (2-pound) eye-of-round roast, trimmed
8 ounces onion, cut in 1/4-inch thick wedges
1 whole head garlic (about 12–16 cloves), peeled only
1 tablespoon canola oil
1/2 cup water

1 Preheat oven to 475°F. Combine the coffee granules, chili powder, salt, and pepper and press the mixture on all sides of the beef. Place the roast in the center of a 13 × 9-inch baking pan, arrange onions and garlic around, and drizzle with oil. Bake 20 minutes, turning the beef and stirring the onion mixture after 10 minutes.

2 Reduce oven temperature to 300°F (do not remove roast from oven). Bake 30 minutes or until a thermometer registers 120°F. Turn off oven. Place the roast on a cutting board and let stand 10 minutes before thinly slicing against the grain. Stir the water into the onion mixture in the pan, scraping the bottom and sides of the pan, and place in oven while the beef is resting. Serve with beef.

EXCHANGES / CHOICES
1 Vegetable
3 Protein, lean
1/2 Fat

BASIC NUTRITIONAL VALUES

Calories	185	**Potassium**	310 mg
Calories from Fat	55	**Total Carbohydrate**	5 g
Total Fat	6.0 g	Dietary Fiber	1 g
Saturated Fat	1.5 g	Sugars	1 g
Trans Fat	0.0 g	**Protein**	27 g
Cholesterol	50 mg	**Phosphorus**	185 mg
Sodium	335 mg		

"2-Minutes-To-Fix" Italian Meatloaf

Serves: 4
Serving Size: 2 slices

1 Preheat oven to 350°F. Meanwhile, combine the beef, oats, stir fry, egg, Worcestershire sauce, oregano, and all but ¼ cup of the pizza sauce in a medium bowl and mix until well blended. Place mixture in a 9 × 5-inch nonstick loaf pan coated with cooking spray.

2 Bake 1 hour or until internal temperature reaches 160°F when tested with a meat thermometer. Spread remaining pizza sauce evenly over all and sprinkle with cheese (if desired) and let stand 5 minutes before cutting into 8 slices.

12 ounces extra-lean (90% lean) ground beef
½ cup quick-cooking oats
½ (14-ounce) package frozen pepper stir-fry, thawed
¼ cup egg substitute
1 teaspoon dried oregano leaves
2 teaspoons Worcestershire sauce
¾ cup pizza sauce
1 tablespoon grated Parmesan cheese (optional)

Cook's Tip: To thaw frozen vegetables quickly, place in a colander and run under cold water 30 seconds, shake off excess liquid.

EXCHANGES / CHOICES
½ Starch
1 Vegetable
3 Protein, lean
1 Fat

BASIC NUTRITIONAL VALUES

Calories	235	**Potassium**	575 mg
Calories from Fat	90	**Total Carbohydrate**	15 g
Total Fat	10.0 g	Dietary Fiber	3 g
Saturated Fat	3.8 g	Sugars	5 g
Trans Fat	0.5 g	**Protein**	21 g
Cholesterol	55 mg	**Phosphorus**	235 mg
Sodium	300 mg		

Chuck and Ale Ragout

2 pounds boneless chuck roast, trimmed of fat, cut into 4–6 chunks*

8 ounces onions, cut in $1/2$-inch thick wedges

12 ounces carrots, cut into 1-inch chunks (or baby carrots)

1 large green bell pepper, cut into 1-inch chunks

1 (14.5-ounce) can no-salt-added stewed tomatoes, drained

1 cup light beer

$1/4$ cup ketchup

1 tablespoon smoked paprika

1 tablespoon balsamic vinegar

2 teaspoons Worcestershire sauce

2 teaspoons dried oregano leaves

1 teaspoon salt

1 Combine all ingredients in a 6-quart slow cooker. Cover and cook on high 5 hours or on low 10 hours.

2 Remove the beef with a slotted spoon, and pull apart larger pieces of beef with two forks. Return to the slow cooker and cook 15 minutes uncovered to thicken slightly. Serve as is in bowls or serve in bowls over $1/2$ cup cooked rice, mashed potatoes, or egg noodles per serving. The beef mixture freezes well.

*Cook's Tip: When purchasing chuck, buy about $1/3$ pound more than you actually need, because the fat has to be removed. Even on the leaner cuts, there's generally some fat that needs to be removed.

EXCHANGES / CHOICES

2 Vegetable
3 Protein, lean
$1/2$ Fat

BASIC NUTRITIONAL VALUES

Calories	220	**Potassium**	735 mg
Calories from Fat	65	**Total Carbohydrate**	13 g
Total Fat	7.0 g	Dietary Fiber	3 g
Saturated Fat	3.1 g	Sugars	8 g
Trans Fat	0.3 g	**Protein**	25 g
Cholesterol	75 mg	**Phosphorus**	270 mg
Sodium	530 mg		

Serves: 4
Serving Size: 3 ounces cooked pork and $\frac{1}{2}$ cup sauce per serving

Pork and Mushroom Ragout

1   Coat both sides of the pork chops in flour. Heat oil in a large skillet over medium-high heat and brown the pork 3 minutes on each side.

2   Top with the remaining ingredients, except parsley. Cover and cook over medium-low heat for 1 hour and 15 minutes or until very tender. Top with parsley. Serve over brown rice, no-yolk egg noodles, or mashed potatoes.

1 pound boneless pork chops, trimmed of fat
$\frac{1}{4}$ **cup** all-purpose flour
2 tablespoons canola oil
8 ounces sliced mushrooms
4 ounces fennel bulb or onion, thinly sliced
3 medium garlic cloves, minced
1 cup dry red wine
$\frac{1}{2}$ **cup** water
$\frac{1}{4}$ **cup** no-salt-added tomato paste
2 tablespoons lemon juice
2 teaspoons sugar
$\frac{1}{2}$ **teaspoon** salt
$\frac{1}{4}$ **teaspoon** black pepper
2 tablespoons chopped fresh Italian parsley

EXCHANGES / CHOICES

1 Carbohydrate
3 Protein, lean
2 Fat

BASIC NUTRITIONAL VALUES

Calories	300	Potassium	810 mg
Calories from Fat	135	**Total Carbohydrate**	17 g
Total Fat	15.0 g	Dietary Fiber	2 g
Saturated Fat	3.1 g	Sugars	6 g
Trans Fat	0.0 g	**Protein**	25 g
Cholesterol	60 mg	**Phosphorus**	265 mg
Sodium	375 mg		

Creamy Pasta Parmesan with Bacon

4 **ounces** uncooked multigrain pasta, such as rotini or linguini

6 **precooked bacon slices**, crumbled, OR **2 ounces** (about 30 pieces) regular turkey pepperoni slices, chopped

2 **cups** loosely packed spinach, coarsely chopped

1 **cup** grape tomatoes, quartered

½ **cup** finely chopped green onion

1 medium garlic clove, minced

¼ **teaspoon** salt

⅛ **teaspoon** dried pepper flakes

4 **teaspoons** grated Parmesan cheese

1 Cook pasta according to package directions.

2 Drain pasta, reserving ⅓ cup pasta water. Place the pasta, reserved water, and the remaining ingredients, except the parmesan in a large bowl. Toss until well blended. Sprinkle with the parmesan.

Cook's Tip: For another flavor addition, add 2–3 tablespoons chopped fresh basil.

EXCHANGES / CHOICES	BASIC NUTRITIONAL VALUES			
1½ Starch	**Calories**	210	**Potassium**	345 mg
1 Protein, high fat	Calories from Fat	65	**Total Carbohydrate**	24 g
	Total Fat	7.0 g	Dietary Fiber	4 g
	Saturated Fat	2.4 g	Sugars	2 g
	Trans Fat	0.0 g	**Protein**	12 g
	Cholesterol	20 mg	**Phosphorus**	165 mg
	Sodium	480 mg		

Shredded Root Beer Pork

SERVES: 8
SERVING SIZE: 1/2 cup pork mixture

1 Place the onions and peppers in the bottom of a 3½ to 4-quart slow cooker. Add the root beer, Worcestershire sauce, soy sauce, and all but 1 tablespoon of the vinegar. Place the pork over all and sprinkle with the allspice, cumin, and pepper flakes.

2 Cover and cook on high for 4 hours or until pork is tender. Shred with a fork in the slow cooker, stir in the remaining vinegar, sugar, and salt. Serve on toasted whole-wheat hamburger buns or on high-fiber, low-carb flour tortillas, if desired.

1 **cup** diced onion
1 ½ **cups** diced green bell pepper
1 **cup** diet root beer
1 **tablespoon** Worcestershire sauce
3 **tablespoons** light soy sauce
3 **tablespoons** balsamic vinegar, divided use
1 ½ **pounds** pork tenderloin
1 **teaspoon** allspice
¾ **teaspoon** ground cumin
¼ **teaspoon** dried pepper flakes
2 **teaspoons** sugar
¼ **teaspoon** salt

EXCHANGES / CHOICES
½ Carbohydrate
2 Protein, lean

BASIC NUTRITIONAL VALUES

Calories	125	**Potassium**	455 mg
Calories from Fat	20	**Total Carbohydrate**	6 g
Total Fat	2.0 g	Dietary Fiber	1 g
Saturated Fat	0.6 g	Sugars	4 g
Trans Fat	0.0 g	**Protein**	19 g
Cholesterol	55 mg	**Phosphorus**	230 mg
Sodium	350 mg		

Smoky Pork Chops with Tomatoes

Serves: 4
Serving Size: 3 ounces cooked pork and 3 tablespoons tomato

¹/₄ **cup** all-purpose flour

1 teaspoon smoked paprika

¹/₂ **teaspoon** dried thyme leaves

¹/₄ **teaspoon** garlic powder

¹/₄ **teaspoon** salt and ¹/₈ **teaspoon** salt, divided use

¹/₂ **teaspoon** black pepper

4 bone-in pork chops, about 5 ounces each

2 tablespoons canola oil

2 medium Roma tomatoes, diced

1. Combine the flour, paprika, thyme, garlic powder, ¹/₄ teaspoon of the salt, and black pepper in a shallow pie pan. Coat the pork chops evenly on both sides.

2. Heat the oil in a large nonstick skillet over medium-high heat and cook 4 minutes on each side or until no longer pink in center. Sprinkle with the diced tomatoes and remaining ¹/₈ teaspoon salt.

EXCHANGES / CHOICES

¹/₂ Carbohydrate
3 Protein, lean
1 ¹/₂ Fat

BASIC NUTRITIONAL VALUES

Calories	230	**Potassium**	360 mg
Calories from Fat	115	**Total Carbohydrate**	6 g
Total Fat	13.0 g	Dietary Fiber	1 g
Saturated Fat	2.7 g	Sugars	1 g
Trans Fat	0.0 g	**Protein**	22 g
Cholesterol	60 mg	**Phosphorus**	140 mg
Sodium	210 mg		

Pork Chops with Tarragon Pepper Sour Cream

Serves: 4

Serving Size: 3 ounces cooked pork and 2 tablespoons aioli

1 Heat the oil in a large nonstick skillet over medium-high heat. Sprinkle both sides of the pork with the onion powder and salt. Cook pork 4 minutes on each side or until slightly pink in center.

2 Meanwhile, stir together the aioli ingredients, except the lime wedges. Serve alongside pork and squeeze lime over all.

2 teaspoons canola oil
4 (4-ounce) boneless center-cut pork chops, trimmed of fat
1/2 teaspoon onion powder
1/4 teaspoon salt

Aioli

1/3 cup fat-free sour cream
2 tablespoons light mayonnaise
1 medium garlic clove, minced
1/4 to 1/2 teaspoon dried tarragon leaves
1/4 teaspoon black pepper, preferably coarsely ground variety
1/8 teaspoon salt
1 medium lime, quartered

EXCHANGES / CHOICES	BASIC NUTRITIONAL VALUES			
1/2 Carbohydrate	**Calories**	215	**Potassium**	340 mg
3 Protein, lean	Calories from Fat	110	**Total Carbohydrate**	5 g
1 Fat	**Total Fat**	12.0 g	Dietary Fiber	0 g
	Saturated Fat	3.4 g	Sugars	1 g
	Trans Fat	0.0 g	**Protein**	21 g
	Cholesterol	55 mg	**Phosphorus**	150 mg
	Sodium	330 mg		

Ham, Potato, and Green Pea Casserole

1 tablespoon canola oil, divided use
6 ounces lean smoked ham, deli sliced and chopped
1 pound red potatoes, thinly sliced
1 medium red bell pepper, diced
1 cup thinly sliced onion
1 cup frozen, thawed green peas
½ teaspoon dried thyme leaves
⅛ teaspoon salt
⅛ teaspoon black pepper
1 ounce reduced-fat blue cheese, crumbled

1   Preheat oven to 350°F. Meanwhile, heat 1 teaspoon of the oil in a medium nonstick skillet over medium-high heat. Brown the ham, stirring occasionally. Stir in the potatoes, bell pepper, onion, peas, thyme, salt, and black pepper and drizzle with the remaining oil.

2   Cover and bake 40 minutes or until potatoes are tender when pierced with a fork. Top with the cheese 3 minutes before the end of cooking time.

Cook's Tip: If time allows, let stand covered 15 minutes to absorb flavors.

Cook's Tip: May transfer the ham and potato mixture to a 2-quart casserole dish instead of baking in the skillet, if desired.

EXCHANGES / CHOICES

1½ Starch
1 Vegetable
1 Protein, lean
½ Fat

BASIC NUTRITIONAL VALUES

Calories	225	**Potassium**	795 mg
Calories from Fat	55	**Total Carbohydrate**	28 g
Total Fat	6.0 g	Dietary Fiber	5 g
Saturated Fat	1.6 g	Sugars	6 g
Trans Fat	0.0 g	**Protein**	14 g
Cholesterol	25 mg	**Phosphorus**	220 mg
Sodium	600 mg		

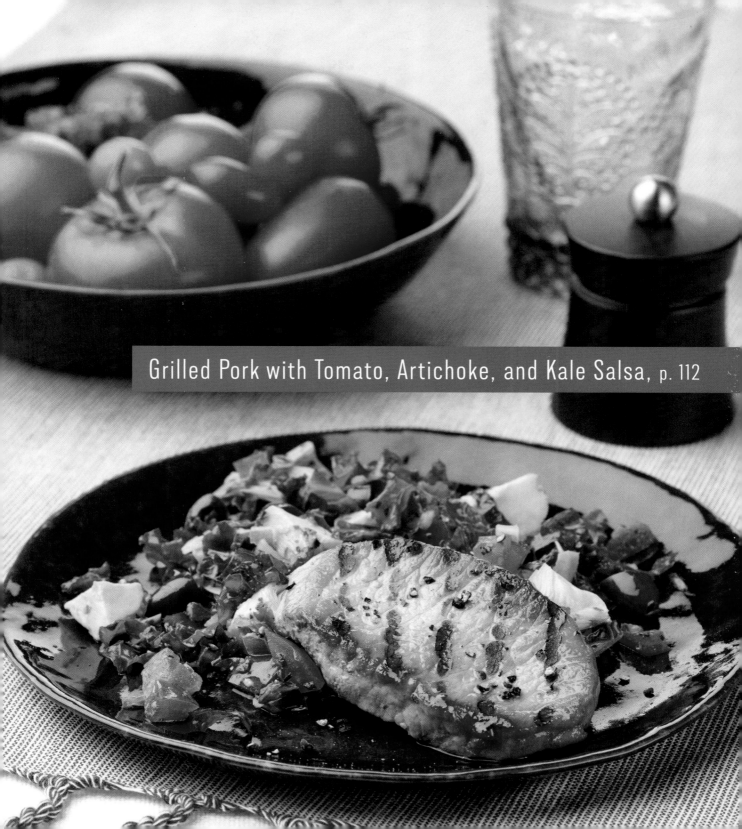

Grilled Pork with Tomato, Artichoke, and Kale Salsa, p. 112

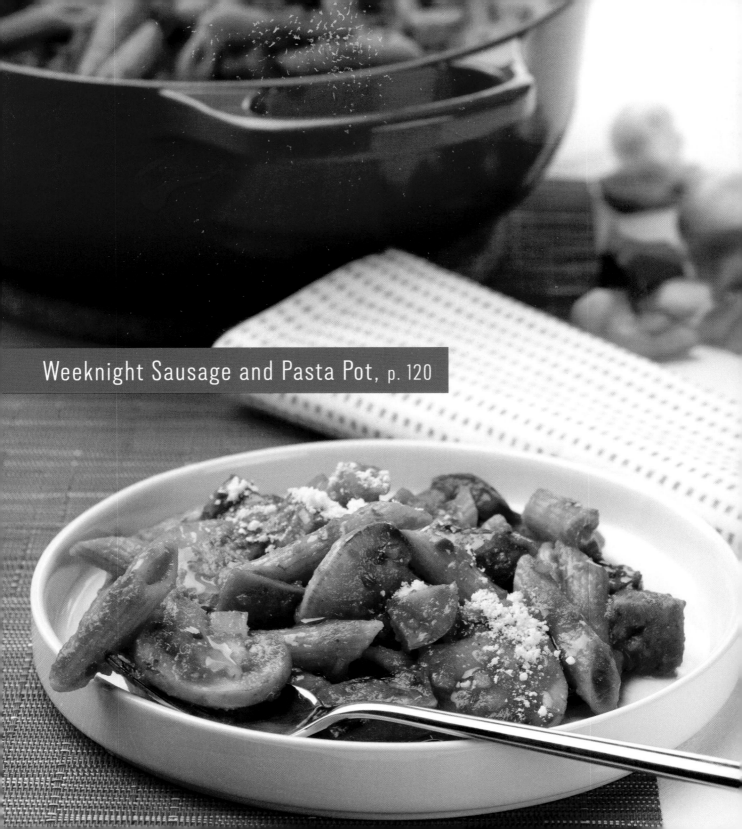

Weeknight Sausage and Pasta Pot, p. 120

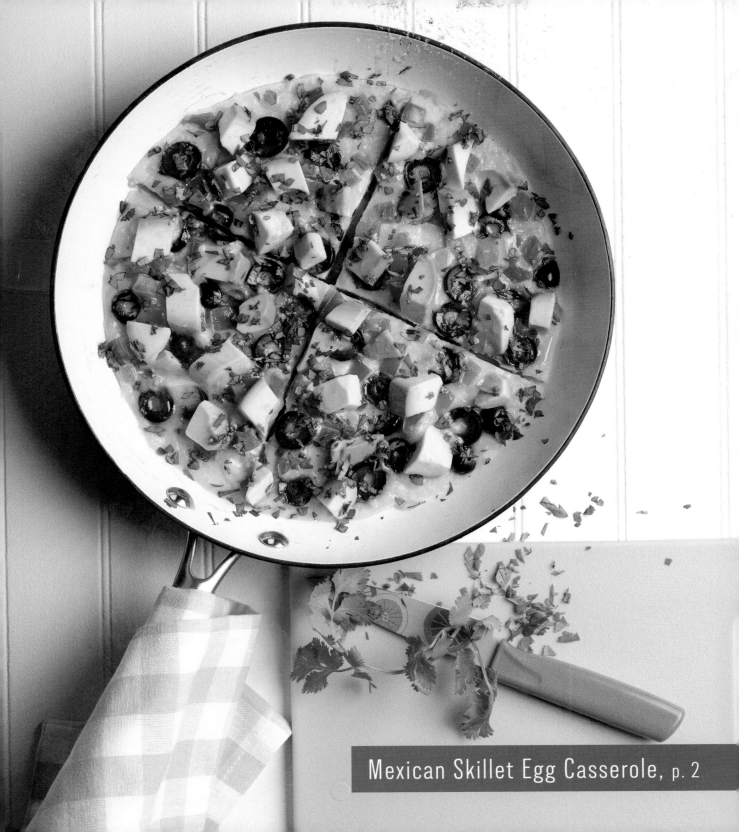

Mexican Skillet Egg Casserole, p. 2

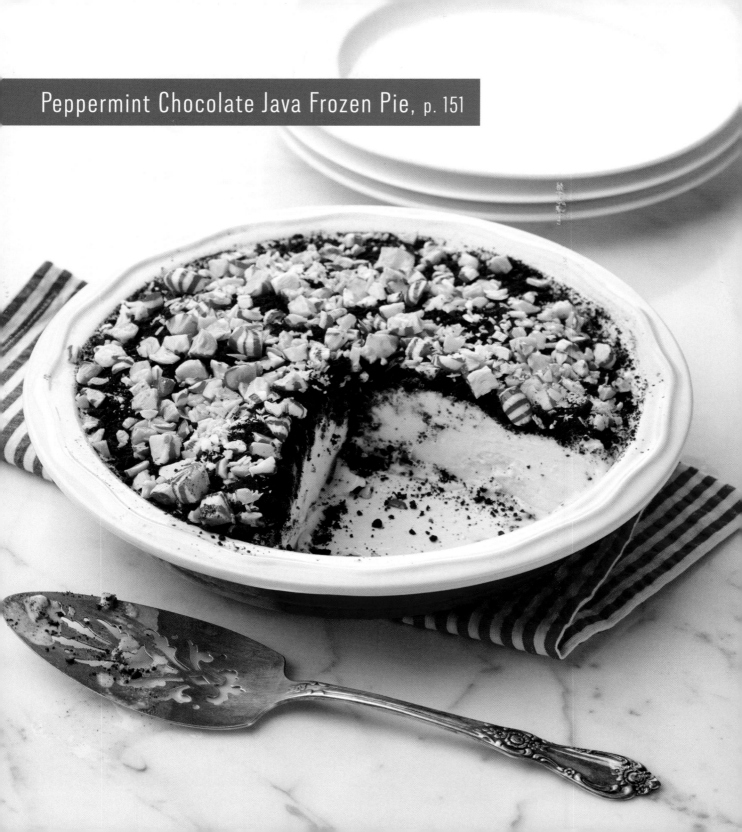

Peppermint Chocolate Java Frozen Pie, p. 151

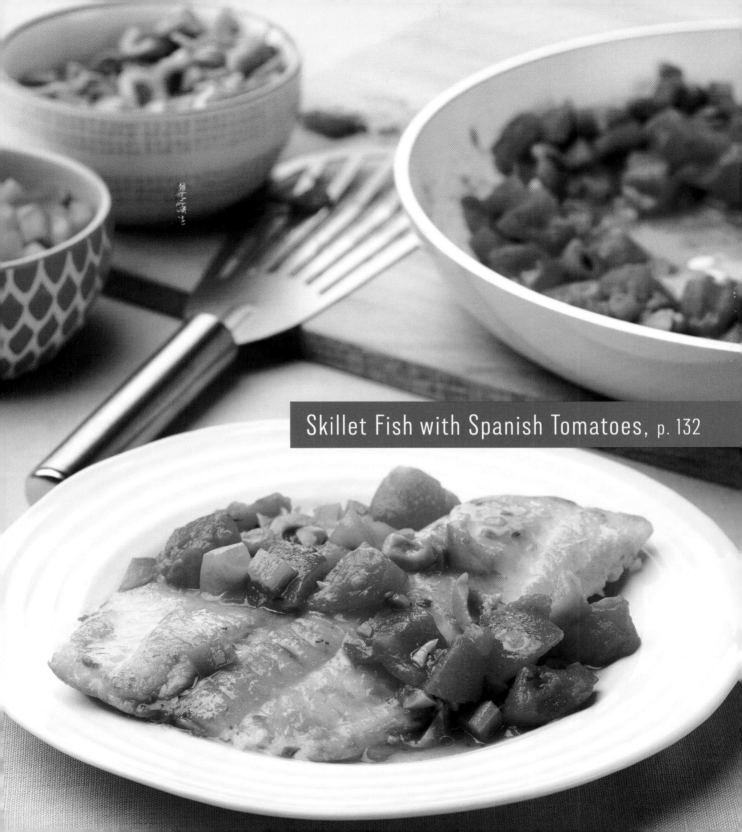

Skillet Fish with Spanish Tomatoes, p. 132

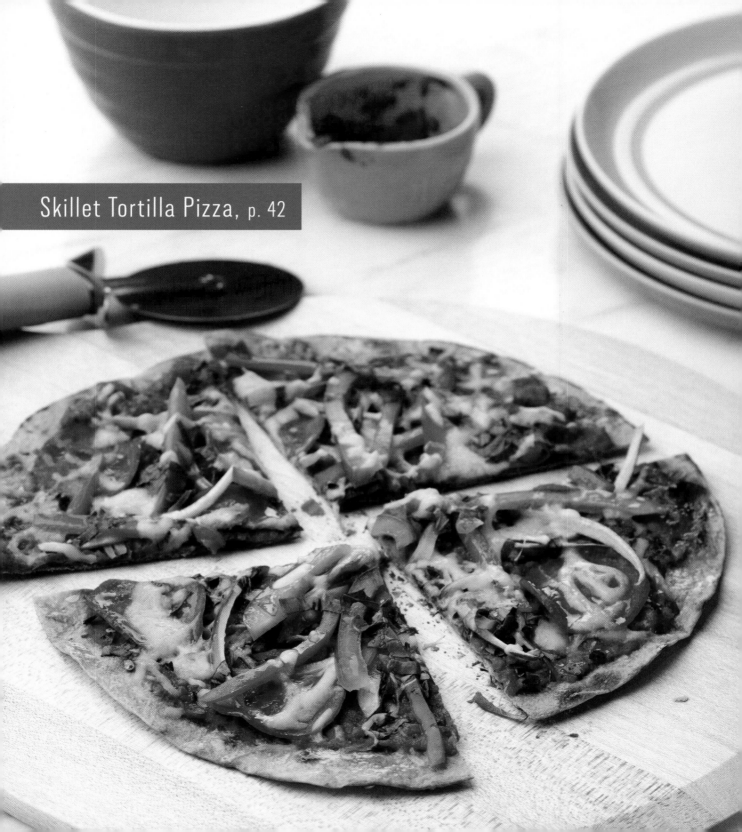

Skillet Tortilla Pizza, p. 42

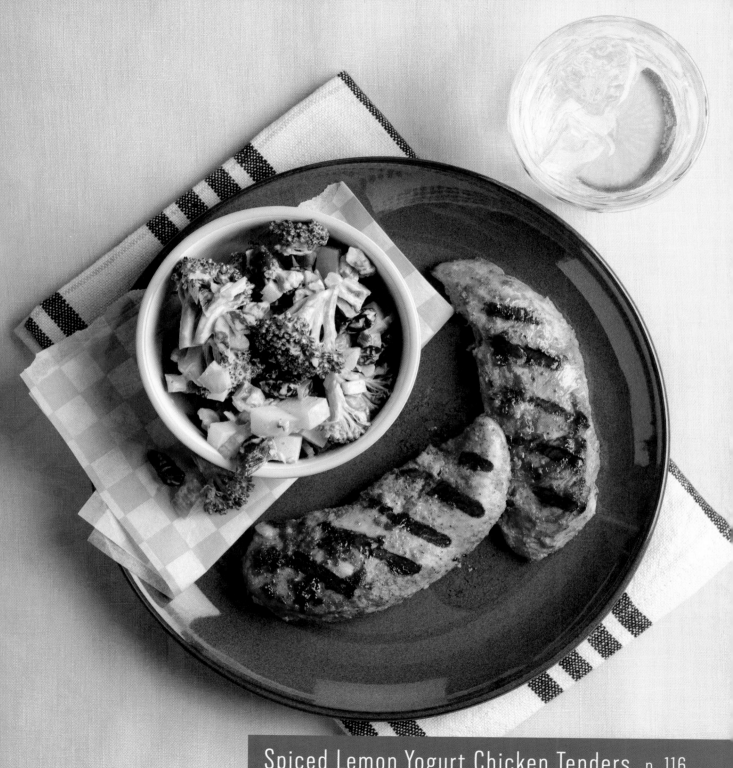

Spiced Lemon Yogurt Chicken Tenders, p. 116

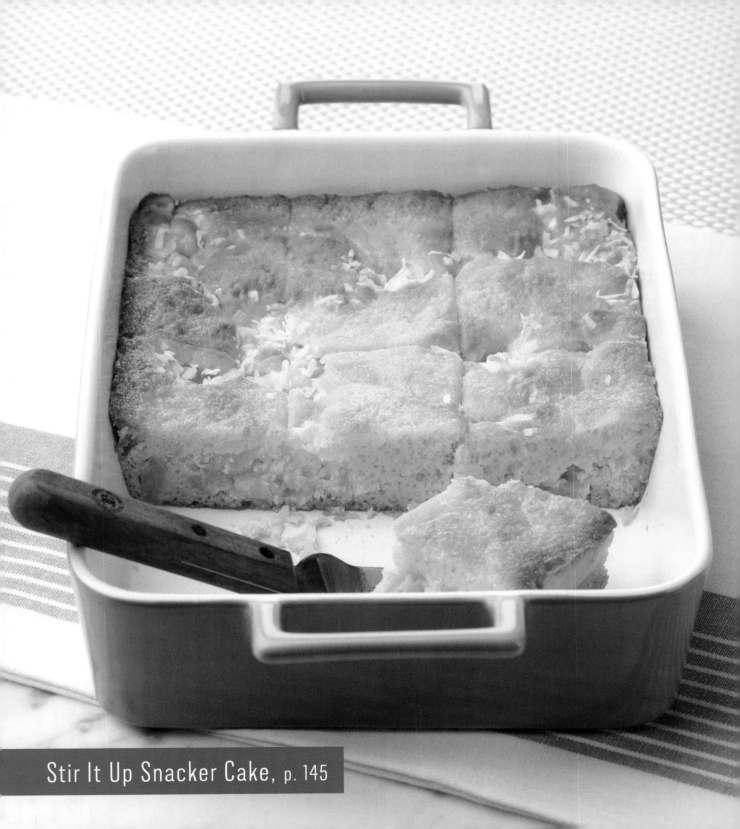

Stir It Up Snacker Cake, p. 145

Sage'd Pork Tenderloin with Roasted Veggies

1 Preheat oven to 425°F. Meanwhile, place the pork and vegetables on a foil-lined baking sheet. Drizzle the vegetables with oil and brush the mustard over the pork. Sprinkle evenly with the remaining ingredients.

2 Bake 25–27 minutes or until pork reaches 145°F. Place pork on cutting board and let stand 3 minutes before slicing. Wrap the veggies in the foil to keep warm and absorb flavors.

1 **pound** pork tenderloin

1 **pound** new potatoes, quartered

1 (4-ounce) onion, cut in $1/2$-inch wedges (about 1 medium)

2 medium carrots, halved lengthwise and cut into 2-inch pieces

1 **tablespoon** extra virgin olive oil

1 $1/2$ **tablespoons** Dijon mustard, preferably coarse-grain variety

$1/2$ **teaspoon** dried sage or poultry seasoning

$1/2$ **teaspoon** garlic powder

$1/2$ **teaspoon** paprika

$1/2$ **teaspoon** salt

$1/4$ **teaspoon** black pepper

EXCHANGES / CHOICES

1 $1/2$ Starch
1 Vegetable
3 Protein, lean

BASIC NUTRITIONAL VALUES

Calories	260	**Potassium**	1010 mg
Calories from Fat	65	**Total Carbohydrate**	25 g
Total Fat	7.0 g	Dietary Fiber	3 g
Saturated Fat	1.5 g	Sugars	4 g
Trans Fat	0.0 g	**Protein**	25 g
Cholesterol	60 mg	**Phosphorus**	290 mg
Sodium	500 mg		

Grilled Pork with Tomato, Artichoke, and Kale Salsa

Pork

4 boneless pork chops
¹/₄ **teaspoon** salt
¹/₄ **teaspoon** black pepper

Salsa

1 **cup** diced tomato
¹/₄ of a 14-ounce can quartered artichoke hearts, chopped
¹/₂ **cup** finely chopped fresh kale
¹/₄ **cup** finely chopped red onion
2 **teaspoons** dried oregano leaves
1 **tablespoon** extra virgin olive oil
2 **teaspoons** cider vinegar
¹/₄ **teaspoon** salt

1 Heat a grill or grill pan coated with cooking spray over medium-high heat. Sprinkle both sides of the pork chops with salt and pepper and cook 4 minutes on each side or until slightly pink in center.

2 Meanwhile, combine salsa ingredients in a medium bowl. Serve with pork.

COOK'S TIP: The salsa is also fun to serve as an appetizer with cucumber rounds or spooned onto Belgian endive.

EXCHANGES / CHOICES	BASIC NUTRITIONAL VALUES			
1 Vegetable	Calories	180	Potassium	460 mg
3 Protein, lean	Calories from Fat	70	**Total Carbohydrate**	8 g
¹/₂ Fat	**Total Fat**	8.0 g	Dietary Fiber	3 g
	Saturated Fat	2.2 g	Sugars	3 g
	Trans Fat	0.0 g	**Protein**	19 g
	Cholesterol	45 mg	**Phosphorus**	145 mg
	Sodium	415 mg		

Serves: 4
Serving Size: 1 mushroom cap plus ¼ cup spinach mixture

1 Preheat oven to 425°F. Meanwhile, combine ½ cup of the spaghetti sauce, spinach, bell pepper, pepperoni, basil, garlic, and pepper flakes in a medium bowl and spoon equal amounts into each mushroom cap.

2 Place mushroom caps on a baking sheet, top with the remaining spaghetti sauce and the cheese. Bake, uncovered, 12–15 minutes or until cheese is melted and slightly browned.

1 cup bottled lower-sodium spaghetti sauce, divided use

1 (10-ounce) package frozen chopped spinach, thawed and squeezed dry

½ cup finely chopped red bell pepper

1 ounce (about 13) turkey pepperoni slices, coarsely chopped

1 tablespoon dried basil leaves

¼ teaspoon garlic powder

⅛ teaspoon dried pepper flakes (optional)

4 large portobello mushroom caps, stems removed, cleaned with damp paper towel

2 ounces shredded part-skim mozzarella cheese

EXCHANGES / CHOICES	BASIC NUTRITIONAL VALUES			
2 Vegetable	**Calories**	130	**Potassium**	705 mg
1 Protein, medium fat	Calories from Fat	55	**Total Carbohydrate**	12 g
	Total Fat	6.0 g	Dietary Fiber	4 g
	Saturated Fat	2.1 g	Sugars	5 g
	Trans Fat	0.0 g	**Protein**	11 g
	Cholesterol	20 mg	**Phosphorus**	190 mg
	Sodium	420 mg		

Italian Sausage, White Bean, and Veggie Soup

SERVES: 4
SERVING SIZE: 1½ cups

1 **teaspoon** canola oil

6 **ounces** mild Italian turkey sausage, casing removed

1 large red bell pepper, chopped

1 (14.5-ounce) can no-salt-added stewed tomatoes

1 (14-ounce) can reduced-sodium chicken broth

1 **cup** water

1 (15-ounce) can no-salt-added navy beans, rinsed and drained

1 **teaspoon** dried oregano leaves

½ **teaspoon** dried fennel (optional)

¼ **teaspoon** salt (optional)

2 **cups** packed chopped kale (about 1½ ounces total)

1 Heat oil in a large saucepan. Add sausage and brown 2–3 minutes, breaking up larger pieces. Stir in remaining ingredients, except the kale. Bring to a boil over high heat, reduce heat to medium low, cover, and cook 20 minutes or until peppers are tender. Remove from heat.

2 Stir in the kale. Let stand 3 minutes to absorb flavors.

COOK'S TIP: There's 70% Vitamin A and 170% Vitamin C of your daily requirements in a single serving!

EXCHANGES / CHOICES

1 Starch
3 Vegetable
1 Protein, lean
½ Fat

BASIC NUTRITIONAL VALUES

Calories	220	**Potassium**	705 mg
Calories from Fat	55	**Total Carbohydrate**	29 g
Total Fat	6.0 g	Dietary Fiber	9 g
Saturated Fat	1.2 g	Sugars	9 g
Trans Fat	0.1 g	**Protein**	16 g
Cholesterol	25 mg	**Phosphorus**	210 mg
Sodium	565 mg		

Chicken, Rice, and Water Chestnut Casserole

SERVES: 4
SERVING SIZE: 1½ cups

1 Preheat oven to 350°F. Meanwhile, combine all the ingredients, except the cheese, almonds, and lemon wedges. Spoon mixture into an 11 × 7-inch baking dish. Sprinkle evenly with the cheese and almonds.

2 Bake, uncovered, for 40 minutes or until heated through and bubbly. Remove from oven and let stand for 10 minutes to absorb flavors. Serve with lemon wedges, if desired.

COOK'S TIP: To thaw frozen vegetables and rice quickly, place in a fine-mesh sieve (not a colander) and run under cold water 20-30 seconds. Shake off excess liquid. If a colander is used, the rice will slip through the larger holes.

2 cups chopped cooked chicken breast meat
2 cups precooked frozen brown rice, thawed
4 ounces sliced mushrooms
1 cup frozen French-cut green beans, thawed
1 (8-ounce) can sliced water chestnuts, drained
4 medium green onions, finely chopped
1 cup 98% fat-free cream of chicken soup
⅓ cup plain, nonfat Greek yogurt
1 teaspoon dried thyme leaves
2 tablespoons grated Parmesan cheese
1 ounce sliced almonds
1 medium lemon, quartered (optional)

EXCHANGES / CHOICES
1½ Starch
½ Carbohydrate
2 Vegetable
3 Protein, lean
½ Fat

BASIC NUTRITIONAL VALUES

Calories	360	**Potassium**	570 mg
Calories from Fat	80	**Total Carbohydrate**	37 g
Total Fat	9.0 g	Dietary Fiber	6 g
Saturated Fat	2.0 g	Sugars	4 g
Trans Fat	0.0 g	**Protein**	31 g
Cholesterol	65 mg	**Phosphorus**	370 mg
Sodium	515 mg		

Spiced Lemon Yogurt Chicken Tenders

8 chicken tenders (or tenderloin),
   rinsed and patted dry (about 1 pound)
1 cup nonfat, plain Greek yogurt
Grated rind and juice of a large lemon
1 tablespoon paprika
1 tablespoon grated gingerroot
1 teaspoon ground cumin
1/2 teaspoon garlic powder
1/2 teaspoon salt
1 medium lemon, quartered (optional)

1   Combine all ingredients, except the lemon quarters, in a gallon resealable plastic bag. Seal tightly and toss back and forth until well coated. Refrigerate 8 hours.

2   Heat a grill pan liberally coated with cooking spray over medium-high heat. Remove chicken from marinade, discarding marinade, and grill 3 minutes on each side or until no longer pink in center. Serve with the quartered lemon, if desired.

EXCHANGES / CHOICES	BASIC NUTRITIONAL VALUES			
1/2 Carbohydrate	**Calories**	175	**Potassium**	345 mg
3 Protein, lean	Calories from Fat	25	**Total Carbohydrate**	5 g
	Total Fat	3.0 g	Dietary Fiber	1 g
	Saturated Fat	0.8 g	Sugars	3 g
	Trans Fat	0.0 g	**Protein**	30 g
	Cholesterol	65 mg	**Phosphorus**	265 mg
	Sodium	375 mg		

Chicken with Mushrooms and Artichoke Hearts

Serves: 4
Serving Size: 3 ounces cooked chicken and ¼ cup artichoke mixture

1   Heat 1 teaspoon of the oil in a large nonstick skillet over medium-high heat. Season chicken on both sides with salt, black pepper, and pepper flakes. Cook 3 minutes on each side or until beginning to brown. Set aside on separate plate. Cover to keep warm.

2   Heat 2 teaspoons of the oil in the skillet. Cook shallots 1 minute, stirring constantly. Stir in mushrooms and cook 4 minutes or until beginning to brown, stirring frequently. Add the broth, artichokes, Worcestershire, lemon juice, and rosemary. Top with chicken and drizzle remaining oil over all. Reduce heat to medium, cook, uncovered, 10 minutes or until chicken is no longer pink in center. Do not stir.

2 tablespoons extra virgin olive oil, divided use
4 (4-ounce) boneless, skinless chicken breasts, rinsed and patted dry
¼ teaspoon salt
¼ teaspoon black pepper
⅛ teaspoon dried pepper flakes
4 medium shallots, thinly sliced
4 ounces sliced mushrooms
1 cup reduced-sodium chicken broth
1 (13.75-ounce) can quartered artichoke hearts, drained
2 teaspoons Worcestershire sauce
1 tablespoon lemon juice
1 teaspoon chopped fresh rosemary

EXCHANGES / CHOICES

3 Vegetable
3 Protein, lean
1 Fat

BASIC NUTRITIONAL VALUES

Calories	255	**Potassium**	610 mg
Calories from Fat	90	**Total Carbohydrate**	14 g
Total Fat	10.0 g	Dietary Fiber	4 g
Saturated Fat	1.8 g	Sugars	2 g
Trans Fat	0.0 g	**Protein**	28 g
Cholesterol	65 mg	**Phosphorus**	265 mg
Sodium	550 mg		

Country-Style Turkey and Gravy Meatloaf

12 ounces ground turkey breast meat
4 ounces Italian turkey sausage, removed from casing
4 ounces sliced mushrooms
½ cup thinly sliced celery
¼ cup chopped parsley, preferably flat-leaf variety
½ cup quick-cooking oats
1 large egg
1 teaspoon dried thyme leaves
2 teaspoons Worcestershire sauce
2 teaspoons Dijon mustard
¾ cup prepared turkey or chicken gravy, preferably the home-style variety

1. Preheat oven to 350°F. Meanwhile, combine all ingredients, except ¼ cup of the gravy, in a 8½ × 4½-inch nonstick loaf pan. Spoon remaining gravy evenly over the top.

2. Bake for 55 minutes or until internal temperature reaches 165°F using a meat thermometer. Remove from oven and let stand on cooling rack 10 minutes before slicing.

EXCHANGES / CHOICES

1 Carbohydrate
4 Protein, lean

BASIC NUTRITIONAL VALUES

Calories	235	**Potassium**	590 mg
Calories from Fat	65	**Total Carbohydrate**	12 g
Total Fat	7.0 g	Dietary Fiber	2 g
Saturated Fat	1.8 g	Sugars	1 g
Trans Fat	0.0 g	**Protein**	30 g
Cholesterol	115 mg	**Phosphorus**	340 mg
Sodium	525 mg		

Herb-Roasted Chicken with Root Vegetables

SERVES: 4
SERVING SIZE: ³/₄ cup chicken and 1¹/₄ cups vegetables

1. Preheat oven to 400°F. Meanwhile, place the chicken (breast side up) on a baking rack in a baking pan. Arrange the vegetables around the chicken. Drizzle the oil evenly over the vegetables only and sprinkle the remaining ingredients evenly over all.

2. Bake 1 hour and 20 minutes or until an instant-read thermometer inserted into the thickest part of the chicken thigh registers 165°F. Let the chicken rest for 20 minutes before slicing. Discard skin.

3 ¹/₂ pounds whole chicken, rinsed and patted dry
1 pound carrots, peeled and cut in thirds crosswise
12 ounces new potatoes, cut in half
1 medium onion (4 ounces), cut into ¹/₂-inch thick wedges
1 tablespoon extra virgin olive oil
1 teaspoon garlic powder
1 teaspoon dried thyme leaves
1 teaspoon dried rosemary
¹/₂ teaspoon paprika
¹/₂ teaspoon black pepper
¹/₂ teaspoon salt

EXCHANGES / CHOICES
1 Starch
2 Vegetable
4 Protein, lean
1 Fat

BASIC NUTRITIONAL VALUES

Calories	345	**Potassium**	970 mg
Calories from Fat	110	**Total Carbohydrate**	27 g
Total Fat	12.0 g	Dietary Fiber	5 g
Saturated Fat	2.7 g	Sugars	7 g
Trans Fat	0.0 g	**Protein**	33 g
Cholesterol	95 mg	**Phosphorus**	295 mg
Sodium	455 mg		

Weeknight Sausage and Pasta Pot

2 tablespoons extra virgin olive oil, divided use
1 large green bell pepper, cut into 1-inch pieces
4 ounces sliced mushrooms
6 ounces multi-grain penne, such as Barilla Plus
1/2 of a 24-ounce container prepared spaghetti sauce
1 1/2 cups water
1 1/2 teaspoons dried oregano leaves, crumbled
1/2 teaspoon dried fennel seed
1/8 teaspoon dried pepper flakes
4 ounces chicken with sun-dried tomatoes sausage, diced
1/2 cup chopped fresh basil
4 teaspoons grated Parmesan cheese

1 Heat 1 teaspoon of the oil over medium-high heat in a Dutch oven. Cook the peppers 4 minutes or until beginning to lightly brown, stirring frequently. Stir in the mushrooms, pasta, spaghetti sauce, water, oregano, fennel seeds, and pepper flakes. Cover, reduce the heat to medium, and cook 14 minutes or until pasta is just tender, stirring occasionally.

2 Remove from heat. Stir in the sausage and basil. Drizzle the remaining oil over all and sprinkle evenly with the cheese. Do not stir. Let stand, uncovered, for 2 minutes to absorb flavors.

EXCHANGES / CHOICES	BASIC NUTRITIONAL VALUES			
2 1/2 Starch	Calories	335	Potassium	615 mg
1 Vegetable	Calories from Fat	110	Total Carbohydrate	41 g
1 Protein, lean	Total Fat	12.0 g	Dietary Fiber	6 g
1 1/2 Fat	Saturated Fat	2.2 g	Sugars	9 g
	Trans Fat	0.0 g	Protein	15 g
	Cholesterol	25 mg	Phosphorus	240 mg
	Sodium	515 mg		

SERVES: 4
SERVING SIZE: 3 ounces cooked chicken and
$^3/_4$ cup rice mixture

1. Heat the oil in a large nonstick skillet over medium-high heat. Brown the chicken on one side, about 2–3 minutes. Turn and brown on the second side. Add the water, picante sauce, and the paprika. Bring to a boil (over medium-high heat), cover, reduce to medium-low, and cook 10 minutes or until chicken is no longer pink in center.

2. Stir in the rice and peas until well blended. Place the chicken on top of the rice, sprinkle the chicken with the cheese and cilantro. Cover and cook 2–3 minutes or until cheese has melted and rice and peas are heated through.

1 teaspoon canola oil
4 (4-ounce) boneless, skinless chicken breasts, rinsed and patted dry
$^1/_3$ **cup** water
$^2/_3$ **cup** mild picante sauce
1 to 1 $^1/_2$ **teaspoons** smoked paprika
1 (8.8-ounce) package cooked whole-grain brown rice
$^3/_4$ **cup** frozen green peas
2 ounces shredded part-skim mozzarella cheese
$^1/_4$ **cup** chopped fresh cilantro

EXCHANGES / CHOICES
1 $^1/_2$ Starch
4 Protein, lean

BASIC NUTRITIONAL VALUES

Calories	290	**Potassium**	400 mg
Calories from Fat	70	**Total Carbohydrate**	24 g
Total Fat	8.0 g	Dietary Fiber	3 g
Saturated Fat	2.4 g	Sugars	2 g
Trans Fat	0.0 g	**Protein**	31 g
Cholesterol	75 mg	**Phosphorus**	330 mg
Sodium	505 mg		

Creole Chicken and Peppers

SERVES: 4
SERVING SIZE: 1 chicken thigh, 1/2 cup pepper mixture, and 1/2 cup rice

1 tablespoon extra virgin olive oil, divided use

4 bone-in chicken thighs, skinned

1/2 (14-ounce) bag frozen pepper stir-fry

1 cup sliced celery

1 dried bay leaf

1/2 teaspoon dried thyme leaves

3/4 cup picante sauce

1 (8.8-ounce) pouch brown rice

1 Heat 1 teaspoon of the oil in a large nonstick skillet over medium-high heat. Brown the chicken on one side, about 5 minutes. Turn and top with the remaining ingredients, except the rice. Bring to a boil, reduce heat to medium-low, cover, and cook 40 minutes or until done.

2 Five minutes before serving, prepare rice according to package directions. Serve chicken mixture over rice.

COOK'S TIP: To remove skin from chicken easily, hold each piece of chicken with a paper towel. Use another paper towel to pull skin away from chicken. Repeat with other chicken pieces and fresh paper towels. The paper towel provides the "traction" needed to hold onto the chicken skin without slipping.

EXCHANGES / CHOICES

1 Starch
1 Vegetable
3 Protein, lean
1 1/2 Fat

BASIC NUTRITIONAL VALUES

Calories	300	**Potassium**	435 mg
Calories from Fat	115	**Total Carbohydrate**	25 g
Total Fat	13.0 g	Dietary Fiber	3 g
Saturated Fat	2.7 g	Sugars	3 g
Trans Fat	0.0 g	**Protein**	23 g
Cholesterol	70 mg	**Phosphorus**	205 mg
Sodium	475 mg		

Creamy Chicken Pasta

Serves: 4
Serving Size: 1 1/2 cups

1 Cook pasta according to package directions and drain.

2 Meanwhile, heat the oil in a large nonstick skillet over medium-high heat. Cook peppers, onion, and mushrooms 6–7 minutes or until peppers are just tender. Stir in the remaining ingredients, except the cheese. Sprinkle evenly with the cheese.

4 ounces multigrain spaghetti noodles
2 teaspoons canola oil
1 1/2 cups chopped red bell pepper
1/2 cup chopped yellow onion
4 ounces sliced mushrooms
2 cups chopped cooked chicken
1 (10.75-ounce) can 98% fat-free cream of chicken soup
1/2 cup nonfat plain Greek yogurt
1/2 teaspoon dried thyme leaves
1/8 teaspoon black pepper
1 tablespoon plus 1 teaspoon grated Parmesan cheese

EXCHANGES / CHOICES

1 Starch
1 Carbohydrate
1 Vegetable
4 Protein, lean
1/2 Fat

BASIC NUTRITIONAL VALUES

Calories	365	**Potassium**	535 mg
Calories from Fat	100	**Total Carbohydrate**	34 g
Total Fat	11.0 g	Dietary Fiber	4 g
Saturated Fat	2.6 g	Sugars	6 g
Trans Fat	0.0 g	**Protein**	31 g
Cholesterol	65 mg	**Phosphorus**	320 mg
Sodium	600 mg		

Chicken with Cilantro-Basil Rice

Serves: 4
Serving Size: 3 ounces cooked chicken and
²/₃ cup rice mixture

2 tablespoons lite soy sauce
4 (4-ounce) boneless, skinless chicken
    breasts, rinsed and patted dry
¹/₈ teaspoon black pepper
1 (8.8-ounce) pouch brown rice
¹/₂ cup frozen green peas, thawed
1 ounce peanuts or slivered almonds,
    coarsely chopped
¹/₄ cup chopped fresh cilantro
2 tablespoons chopped fresh basil
2 tablespoons lime juice
¹/₂ teaspoon grated lime zest
2 teaspoons canola oil
¹/₈ teaspoon dried pepper flakes
¹/₄ teaspoon salt

1   Spoon the soy sauce over the chicken, turning several times to coat. Heat the grill or grill pan coated with cooking spray over medium-high heat. Remove the chicken from the marinade, discarding marinade. Sprinkle with black pepper and grill 5 minutes on each side or until no longer pink in center.

2   Meanwhile, cook the rice according to package directions. Place in a bowl and toss with the remaining ingredients. Serve with the chicken on the side.

EXCHANGES / CHOICES	BASIC NUTRITIONAL VALUES			
1 ¹/₂ Starch	**Calories**	290	**Potassium**	330 mg
4 Protein, lean	Calories from Fat	90	**Total Carbohydrate**	22 g
	Total Fat	10.0 g	Dietary Fiber	3 g
	Saturated Fat	1.5 g	Sugars	1 g
	Trans Fat	0.0 g	**Protein**	29 g
	Cholesterol	65 mg	**Phosphorus**	280 mg
	Sodium	315 mg		

Ground Turkey Patty Pilers

SERVES: 4
SERVING SIZE: 3 ounces cooked turkey patty and ½ cup topping

1 Heat the oil in a large nonstick skillet over medium-high heat. Cook the bell pepper 3 minutes or until just beginning to lightly brown on edges, stirring occasionally. Add the mushrooms and cook 4 minutes or until soft, stirring occasionally. Set aside.

2 Combine the ground turkey, sausage, basil, fennel, and pepper flakes. Shape into 4 hamburger patties (about 4 inches in diameter and ½-inch thick). Cook in skillet 4 minutes, turn, and top with the peppers and mushrooms. Drizzle the wine and spaghetti sauce over all and sprinkle evenly with the salt. Reduce heat to medium-low, cover, and cook for 4 minutes or until turkey is no longer pink in center. Top with mozzarella and sprinkle evenly with the Parmesan cheese.

COOK'S TIP: When buying ground turkey, be sure you're buying ground turkey breast, not regular ground turkey that is much higher in fat.

1 teaspoon canola oil
1 medium green bell pepper, thinly sliced
4 ounces sliced mushrooms
12 ounces ground turkey breast meat
4 ounces hot or mild Italian turkey sausage, casing removed and chopped into small pieces
2 teaspoons dried basil leaves
½ teaspoon dried fennel seed
⅛ teaspoon dried pepper flakes (optional)
2 tablespoons dry red wine
⅔ cup bottled spaghetti sauce
⅛ teaspoon salt
1 ounce grated mozzarella cheese
4 teaspoons grated Parmesan cheese

EXCHANGES / CHOICES
½ Carbohydrate
4 Protein, lean

BASIC NUTRITIONAL VALUES

Calories	220	**Potassium**	600 mg
Calories from Fat	70	**Total Carbohydrate**	7 g
Total Fat	8.0 g	Dietary Fiber	2 g
Saturated Fat	2.3 g	Sugars	4 g
Trans Fat	0.1 g	**Protein**	30 g
Cholesterol	70 mg	**Phosphorus**	325 mg
Sodium	560 mg		

Grilled Tuna Fillets with Caprese Relish

SERVES: 4
SERVING SIZE: 3 ounces cooked fillets and ¼ cup relish

Relish

4 ounces plum tomatoes, diced

1 ounce reduced-fat mozzarella string cheese, diced

2 tablespoons chopped fresh basil

1 teaspoon grated lemon rind

1–2 tablespoons fresh lemon juice

1 tablespoon extra virgin olive oil

1 medium garlic clove, minced

¼ teaspoon salt

⅛ teaspoon dried pepper flakes

Fillets

4 (4-ounce) tuna fillets

2 teaspoons canola oil or extra virgin olive oil

¼ teaspoon salt

¼ teaspoon black pepper

1 Combine the relish ingredients in a small bowl and set aside.

2 Heat a grill pan coated with cooking spray over high heat. Brush both sides of the fish with the remaining 2 teaspoons oil and sprinkle with the salt and pepper. Cook 1½ to 2 minutes on each side or to desired doneness. Serve with relish on the side.

COOK'S TIP: Tuna should be cooked very rare, otherwise it will be tough and dry.

EXCHANGES / CHOICES

4 Protein, lean
1½ Fat

BASIC NUTRITIONAL VALUES

Calories	240	**Potassium**	380 mg
Calories from Fat	110	**Total Carbohydrate**	2 g
Total Fat	12.0 g	Dietary Fiber	0 g
Saturated Fat	24 g	Sugars	1 g
Trans Fat	0.0 g	**Protein**	30 g
Cholesterol	45 mg	**Phosphorus**	345 mg
Sodium	385 mg		

Grilled Halibut with Banana-Mango Lime Salsa Salad

SERVES: 4
SERVING SIZE: 3 ounces cooked fish and ½ cup salad

1 Preheat a grill or grill pan over medium-high heat. Brush the fish with the oil and sprinkle evenly with salt, cumin, and black pepper. Cook 4 minutes on each side or until opaque in center.

2 Meanwhile, combine the salad ingredients and toss gently. Serve fish with lime wedges and salad on the side.

4 (4-ounce) halibut (or cod) fillets, rinsed and pat dry
1 tablespoon canola oil
¼ teaspoon salt
¼ teaspoon ground cumin
¼ teaspoon black pepper

Salad
1 cup diced mango
½ cup diced banana
1 medium jalapeño, seeded and finely chopped
2 tablespoons finely chopped red onion
2 tablespoons chopped fresh cilantro
2 teaspoons grated lime rind
2 tablespoons lime juice
1 tablespoon honey

EXCHANGES / CHOICES	BASIC NUTRITIONAL VALUES			
1 Fruit	**Calories**	225	**Potassium**	710 mg
3 Protein, lean	Calories from Fat	55	**Total Carbohydrate**	18 g
½ Fat	**Total Fat**	6.0 g	Dietary Fiber	2 g
	Saturated Fat	0.7 g	Sugars	14 g
	Trans Fat	0.0 g	**Protein**	25 g
	Cholesterol	35 mg	**Phosphorus**	270 mg
	Sodium	210 mg		

Louisiana Shrimp and Red Pepper Pasta

Serves: 4
Serving Size: 1 1/2 cups

6 **ounces** multigrain rotini pasta

8 **ounces** raw peeled shrimp

2 **tablespoons** extra virgin olive oil, divided use

1 1/2 **cups** thinly sliced red bell pepper

1 1/2 **cups** diced onion

1 **cup** thinly sliced celery

1/2 **cup** finely chopped fresh parsley

1 **tablespoon** Louisiana hot sauce

1/4 **teaspoon** salt

1 medium garlic clove, minced

2 **tablespoons** lower-fat (<50% vegetable oil) margarine-type spread

1 medium lemon, quartered

1 Cook pasta according to package directions, adding the shrimp 4 minutes before end of cooking time. Drain.

2 Meanwhile, heat 2 teaspoons of the oil in a large nonstick skillet. Cook the peppers, onions, and celery 4 minutes or until just tender and beginning to lightly brown. Add drained pasta mixture and remaining ingredients, except lemon wedges. Toss until well blended. Serve with lemon wedges.

EXCHANGES / CHOICES

2 Starch
2 Vegetable
1 Protein, lean
1 1/2 Fat

BASIC NUTRITIONAL VALUES

Calories	325	**Potassium**	450 mg
Calories from Fat	110	**Total Carbohydrate**	39 g
Total Fat	12.0 g	Dietary Fiber	5 g
Saturated Fat	1.9 g	Sugars	6 g
Trans Fat	0.0 g	**Protein**	17 g
Cholesterol	75 mg	**Phosphorus**	260 mg
Sodium	590 mg		

Roast Salmon with Dilled Yogurt Tomatoes

1 Preheat oven to 350°F. Meanwhile, place the salmon, skin side down, on a foil-lined baking sheet. Brush the oil over the fish and sprinkle with the oregano, $^1/_8$ teaspoon salt, and $^1/_8$ teaspoon black pepper. Combine the remaining ingredients, except the tomatoes, in a small bowl.

2 Bake the salmon 18–20 minutes or until opaque in center. Serve the caper mixture on top of the tomatoes and alongside the salmon.

1 $^1/_4$ **pounds** salmon fillet
2 **teaspoons** canola oil
$^1/_2$ **teaspoon** dried oregano leaves
$^1/_4$ **teaspoon** salt, divided use
$^1/_4$ **teaspoon** black pepper, divided use
$^1/_4$ **cup** peeled and finely chopped cucumber
1 $^1/_2$ **tablespoons** drained capers
$^1/_3$ **cup** Greek nonfat yogurt
1 **tablespoon** light mayonnaise
1 **tablespoon** chopped fresh dill
2 medium tomatoes, sliced

EXCHANGES / CHOICES

1 Vegetable
4 Protein, lean
2 Fat

BASIC NUTRITIONAL VALUES

Calories	305	**Potassium**	650 mg
Calories from Fat	145	**Total Carbohydrate**	5 g
Total Fat	16.0 g	Dietary Fiber	1 g
Saturated Fat	2.5 g	Sugars	3 g
Trans Fat	0.0 g	**Protein**	34 g
Cholesterol	100 mg	**Phosphorus**	365 mg
Sodium	350 mg		

Panko Parmesan Baked Tilapia

Serves: 4

Serving Size: 1 fillet

4 6-ounce tilapia fillets, rinsed and patted dry

2 tablespoons light mayonnaise

⅓ cup panko breadcrumbs

1 tablespoon grated lemon zest

¼ cup grated Parmesan cheese

2 tablespoon finely chopped fresh parsley

1 tablespoon canola oil

½ teaspoon dried oregano leaves

½ teaspoon paprika

¼ teaspoon salt

8 medium tomato slices

1 Preheat oven to 400°F. Meanwhile place the tilapia on a foil-lined baking sheet coated with cooking spray and brush the mayonnaise over fish. Combine the remaining ingredients in a small bowl. Using a fork, stir to a crumble texture, and mound on top of the fillets.

2 Bake 18–20 minutes or until fish is opaque in center. Serve with 2 slices of tomato on the side.

EXCHANGES / CHOICES

½ Carbohydrate
5 Protein, lean

BASIC NUTRITIONAL VALUES

Calories	260	**Potassium**	610 mg
Calories from Fat	90	**Total Carbohydrate**	7 g
Total Fat	10.0 g	Dietary Fiber	1 g
Saturated Fat	2.5 g	Sugars	2 g
Trans Fat	0.0 g	**Protein**	36 g
Cholesterol	75 mg	**Phosphorus**	310 mg
Sodium	360 mg		

Serves: 4
Serving Size: 3 ounces cooked fish fillet, 4 ounces asparagus spears, and about 4 teaspoons margarine mixture

Baked Cod with Buttery Lemon Parsley

1 Preheat oven to 425°F. Meanwhile, coat 2 foil-lined baking sheets with cooking spray. Arrange the fish on one baking sheet and the asparagus on the other in a single layer. Coat all with cooking spray. Sprinkle the fish with the seafood seasoning and black pepper and sprinkle the asparagus with the salt. Bake 14 minutes or until fish flakes with a fork.

2 Combine the remaining ingredients, except the lemon quarters, in a small bowl. Serve asparagus alongside fish. Squeeze lemon juice over all and top fish with the margarine mixture.

4 (4-ounce) cod fillets, rinsed and patted dry
1 pound asparagus spears, ends trimmed
1/2 teaspoon seafood seasoning, such as Old Bay
1/8 teaspoon black pepper
1/4 teaspoon salt
1/4 cup lower-fat (<50% vegetable oil) margarine-type spread
2 teaspoons grated lemon rind
2 tablespoons finely chopped fresh parsley
1 medium lemon, quartered

EXCHANGES / CHOICES

3 Protein, lean
1/2 Fat

BASIC NUTRITIONAL VALUES

Calories	160	Potassium	370 mg
Calories from Fat	55	Total Carbohydrate	4 g
Total Fat	6.0 g	Dietary Fiber	1 g
Saturated Fat	1.3 g	Sugars	1 g
Trans Fat	0.0 g	Protein	22 g
Cholesterol	50 mg	Phosphorus	155 mg
Sodium	395 mg		

Skillet Fish with Spanish Tomatoes

Serves: 4
Serving Size: 3 ounces cooked fish and 1/2 cup tomato mixture

1 tablespoon extra virgin olive oil, divided use

4 (4-ounce) tilapia fillets or any other lean white fish fillet, rinsed and patted dry

1 (14.5-ounce) can no-salt-added diced tomatoes

1/2 cup diced green bell pepper

1/2 cup coarsely chopped pimiento-stuffed green olives (about 12 olives)

1/2 teaspoon dried oregano leaves

1/8 teaspoon salt

1. Heat 1 teaspoon oil in a large nonstick skillet over medium-high heat. Cook fish 5 minutes on each side or until it flakes with a fork. Set aside on separate plate.

2. Add the remaining ingredients to the skillet, reduce the heat to medium, cover, and cook 5 minutes or until thickened slightly. Spoon over fish. Serve in shallow bowls, if desired.

Cook's Tip: Serving this recipe in shallow bowls helps to "manage" the juicy tomato mixture.

EXCHANGES / CHOICES

1 Vegetable
3 Protein, lean

BASIC NUTRITIONAL VALUES

Calories	175	**Potassium**	555 mg
Calories from Fat	65	**Total Carbohydrate**	5 g
Total Fat	7.0 g	Dietary Fiber	2 g
Saturated Fat	1.5 g	Sugars	3 g
Trans Fat	0.0 g	**Protein**	23 g
Cholesterol	50 mg	**Phosphorus**	195 mg
Sodium	300 mg		

Rosemary and Thyme Fish Fillets

Serves: 4
Serving Size: 3 ounce fish fillet

1 Heat oil in a large nonstick skillet over medium heat. Add fish, cook 3 minutes, turn, and sprinkle the thyme, rosemary, garlic powder, salt, and pepper over all. Cook 3 minutes or until flaky. Remove fish and set aside on separate plate.

2 Remove skillet from heat. Add margarine and lemon juice, stirring until margarine melts. Serve sauce over fish.

1 ½ **tablespoons** extra virgin olive oil
4 (4-ounce) fish fillets, rinsed and patted dry
½ **teaspoon** dried thyme leaves
¼ **teaspoon** dried rosemary
⅛ **teaspoon** garlic powder
¼ **teaspoon** salt
¼ **teaspoon** black pepper
2 **teaspoons** lower-fat (<50% vegetable oil) margarine-type spread
1 **teaspoon** fresh lemon juice

EXCHANGES / CHOICES

3 Protein, lean
½ Fat

BASIC NUTRITIONAL VALUES

Calories	165	**Potassium**	465 mg
Calories from Fat	65	**Total Carbohydrate**	0 g
Total Fat	7.0 g	Dietary Fiber	0 g
Saturated Fat	1.2 g	Sugars	0 g
Trans Fat	0.0 g	**Protein**	23 g
Cholesterol	40 mg	**Phosphorus**	180 mg
Sodium	210 mg		

Garden Vegetable and Pine Nut Penne

SERVES: 4
SERVING SIZE: 1½ cups

4 ounces whole-grain or multigrain penne pasta

3 cups fresh or frozen, thawed broccoli florets

1 large red bell pepper, thinly sliced

2 ounces (½ cup) pine nuts or slivered almonds, preferably toasted

2 medium garlic cloves, minced

2 teaspoons canola oil

¾ teaspoon salt

1 ounce (¼ cup) grated Parmesan cheese

1   Cook the pasta according to package directions, adding the broccoli and bell pepper during the last 4 minutes of cooking. Drain pasta mixture, shaking off excess liquid.

2   Place pasta mixture in a large bowl with the remaining ingredients, except the cheese, and toss until well blended. Sprinkle with cheese.

COOK'S TIP: Explodes with nutritional benefits . . . 60% of your daily requirement of Vitamin A and 210% of Vitamin C.

EXCHANGES / CHOICES

1½ Starch
1 Vegetable
3 Fat

BASIC NUTRITIONAL VALUES

Calories	280	**Potassium**	395 mg
Calories from Fat	135	**Total Carbohydrate**	30 g
Total Fat	15.0 g	Dietary Fiber	6 g
Saturated Fat	2.1 g	Sugars	5 g
Trans Fat	0.0 g	**Protein**	10 g
Cholesterol	5 mg	**Phosphorus**	230 mg
Sodium	570 mg		

Chunky Country Veggie Sauce

Serves: 6
Serving Size: $^2/_3$ cup

1 Combine the bell pepper, mushrooms, squash, onions, carrots, garlic, and tomatoes in a large saucepan. Bring to a boil over medium-high heat, reduce heat to medium-low, cover, and cook 30 minutes or until thickened and onions are very tender.

2 Remove from heat, stir in the remaining ingredients, and let stand, covered, 5 minutes to develop flavors. Serve over multigrain pasta, brown rice, or baked potatoes. Serve over grilled chicken or fish, if desired.

1 large red bell pepper, coarsely chopped
4 ounces sliced mushrooms
1 medium yellow squash, quartered lengthwise and coarsely chopped
1 cup diced onion
$^1/_2$ **cup** frozen sliced carrots
2 medium garlic cloves, minced
1 (14.5-ounce) can no-salt-added stewed tomatoes
24 kalamata olives, coarsely chopped
$^1/_3$ **cup** chopped fresh basil
1 tablespoon extra virgin olive oil
1 teaspoon chopped fresh rosemary
$^1/_2$ **teaspoon** salt

EXCHANGES / CHOICES	BASIC NUTRITIONAL VALUES			
3 Vegetable	**Calories**	100	**Potassium**	450 mg
1 Fat	Calories from Fat	55	**Total Carbohydrate**	13 g
	Total Fat	6.0 g	Dietary Fiber	3 g
	Saturated Fat	0.6 g	Sugars	8 g
	Trans Fat	0.0 g	**Protein**	2 g
	Cholesterol	0 mg	**Phosphorus**	65 mg
	Sodium	350 mg		

Mexican Rice and Bean Skillet

1 **teaspoon** canola oil

¹/₂ **cup** chopped onions

1 (15.5-ounce) can dark kidney beans, drained and rinsed

1 (1.25-ounce) package 30% less sodium taco seasoning

1 (14.5-ounce) can no-salt-added stewed tomatoes

1 (4-ounce) can chopped mild green chilies

1 **cup** water

³/₄ **cup** instant brown rice

1 ¹/₂ **teaspoons** sugar

2 **ounces** reduced-fat sharp cheddar cheese

1   Heat the oil in a large nonstick skillet over medium-high heat. Cook the onions 4 minutes or until soft, stirring frequently. Add the remaining ingredients, except the cheese, reduce heat to medium, cover, and cook 12 minutes or until rice is tender.

2   Remove from heat and top with cheese.

EXCHANGES / CHOICES

2 ¹/₂ Starch
¹/₂ Carbohydrate
1 Vegetable
1 Protein, lean

BASIC NUTRITIONAL VALUES

Calories	275	**Potassium**	625 mg
Calories from Fat	35	**Total Carbohydrate**	50 g
Total Fat	4.0 g	Dietary Fiber	7 g
Saturated Fat	1.4 g	Sugars	10 g
Trans Fat	0.0 g	**Protein**	13 g
Cholesterol	5 mg	**Phosphorus**	290 mg
Sodium	595 mg		

Portobello Burgers with Blue Cheese Garlic Spread

SERVES: 4
SERVING SIZE: 1 burger plus about 1 1/2 tablespoons cheese spread

1 Preheat grill or grill pan coated with cooking spray over medium-high heat. Coat both sides of the mushrooms with cooking spray and grill 4 minutes on each side or until mushrooms are just tender. Add sandwich rolls and cook 30 seconds on each side.

2 Meanwhile, combine cheese, mayonnaise, milk, garlic, basil, salt, and pepper in a small bowl, mashing with a fork to break up larger pieces of cheese. Stir until well blended. Spoon equal amounts of the blue cheese mixture on bottom half of each roll. Top each serving with mushroom, lettuce, and onion and top with top halves of rolls.

4 medium to large Portobello caps, wiped clean with damp towel
4 onion sandwich rolls
1/4 **cup** crumbled reduced-fat blue cheese
3 **tablespoons** light mayonnaise
1 **tablespoon** fat-free milk
1 medium garlic clove, minced
3/4 **teaspoon** dried basil leaves
1/4 **teaspoon** salt
1/4 **teaspoon** black pepper
4 romaine lettuce leaves
4 **slices** red onion

EXCHANGES / CHOICES

2 Starch
1 Vegetable
1 Fat

BASIC NUTRITIONAL VALUES

Calories	220	**Potassium**	410 mg
Calories from Fat	55	**Total Carbohydrate**	32 g
Total Fat	6.0 g	Dietary Fiber	2 g
Saturated Fat	1.7 g	Sugars	6 g
Trans Fat	0.0 g	**Protein**	9 g
Cholesterol	5 mg	**Phosphorus**	170 mg
Sodium	595 mg		

Farro, Edamame, and Dried Cranberry Salad

¾ cup pearled farro
1 cup shelled edamame
½ cup chopped celery
⅓ cup diced red onion
2 ounces chopped walnuts
¼ cup dried cranberries
¼ cup chopped fresh cilantro or parsley
2 teaspoons grated lemon zest
1 tablespoon lemon juice
1 tablespoon sugar
2 tablespoons canola oil

1 Cook farro according to package directions, drain in fine-mesh sieve, run under cold water to quickly cool, and shake off excess liquid.

2 Place in bowl with remaining ingredients. Toss well.

EXCHANGES / CHOICES

2 Starch
½ Fruit
1 Vegetable
1 Protein, lean
2½ Fat

BASIC NUTRITIONAL VALUES

Calories	375	**Potassium**	425 mg
Calories from Fat	170	**Total Carbohydrate**	44 g
Total Fat	19.0 g	Dietary Fiber	8 g
Saturated Fat	1.8 g	Sugars	10 g
Trans Fat	0.0 g	**Protein**	12 g
Cholesterol	0 mg	**Phosphorus**	250 mg
Sodium	15 mg		

Kale, Feta & White Bean Pizza

Serves: 6
Serving Size: 1 slice

1 Preheat oven to 450°F. Place pizza crust on a baking sheet and bake 6 minutes.

2 Top with the remaining ingredients in the order listed and bake 8 minutes or until crust is golden. Cut into 6 slices.

1 (12-inch) 100% whole-wheat pizza crust
1/3 **cup** pizza sauce
1 **teaspoon** dried oregano leaves
1/8 **teaspoon** dried pepper flakes
1 **cup** thinly sliced red bell pepper
1/2 **cup** thinly sliced red onion
1/2 (15-ounce) can no-salt-added navy beans, drained and rinsed
3/4 **cup** chopped kale
1/2 **cup** crumbled fat-free feta cheese

EXCHANGES / CHOICES
2 Starch
1 Protein, lean

BASIC NUTRITIONAL VALUES

Calories	180	**Potassium**	325 mg
Calories from Fat	25	**Total Carbohydrate**	32 g
Total Fat	3.0 g	Dietary Fiber	7 g
Saturated Fat	1.1 g	Sugars	4 g
Trans Fat	0.0 g	**Protein**	10 g
Cholesterol	0 mg	**Phosphorus**	190 mg
Sodium	435 mg		

DESSERTS

Mango Pineapple Sorbet

8 ounces frozen chopped mango

$^1/_2$ (8-ounce) can unsweetened crushed pineapple

1 $^1/_2$ **tablespoons** fresh lime juice

1 Combine all ingredients in a blender and puree until smooth.

2 Serve immediately as a sorbet or spoon equal amounts into 4 popsicle molds and freeze until firm, about 4 hours.

EXCHANGES / CHOICES

1 Fruit

BASIC NUTRITIONAL VALUES

Calories	50	**Potassium**	130 mg
Calories from Fat	0	**Total Carbohydrate**	14 g
Total Fat	0.0 g	Dietary Fiber	1 g
Saturated Fat	0.0 g	Sugars	11 g
Trans Fat	0.0 g	**Protein**	0 g
Cholesterol	0 mg	**Phosphorus**	10 mg
Sodium	0 mg		

SERVES: 4
SERVING SIZE: $^1/_3$ cup

1   Place all ingredients in a blender and puree until smooth.

2   Pour equal amounts into four ramekins and freeze 1 hour
    for a soft-serve dessert or spoon into 4 popsicle molds
    and freeze 4 hours or until frozen.

1 ripe medium banana
3 tablespoons fat-free half and half
1 teaspoon vanilla extract
1 tablespoon packed dark brown sugar
1 tablespoon plus 1 teaspoon mini
    chocolate chips
2 tablespoons reduced-fat peanut butter
$^3/_4$ cup ice cubes

**EXCHANGES /
CHOICES**

1 Carbohydrate
1 Fat

BASIC NUTRITIONAL VALUES

Calories	120	**Potassium**	225 mg
Calories from Fat	40	**Total Carbohydrate**	18 g
Total Fat	4.5 g	Dietary Fiber	2 g
Saturated Fat	1.4 g	Sugars	12 g
Trans Fat	0.0 g	**Protein**	3 g
Cholesterol	0 mg	**Phosphorus**	60 mg
Sodium	55 mg		

Peach-Pineapple Cobbler

1 **cup** all-purpose flour

$^1/_4$ **cup** granulated sugar

3 **tablespoons** ground flax meal

1 $^1/_2$ **teaspoons** baking powder

$^1/_4$ **teaspoon** salt

1 **large** egg

$^1/_3$ **cup** nonfat plain Greek yogurt

3 **tablespoons** canola oil

1 **teaspoon** vanilla extract

1 (15-ounce) can sliced peaches in extra-
light syrup, drained, reserving juices

8-ounce can pineapple tidbits in own
juice, drained

1 Preheat oven 375°F. Meanwhile, stir together the flour, sugar, flax meal, baking powder, salt, egg, yogurt, oil, vanilla, and peach juice in a medium bowl and pour into a 11 × 7-inch baking pan. Arrange the fruit on top.

2 Bake for 30 minutes or until wooden pick inserted in center comes out clean.

EXCHANGES / CHOICES	BASIC NUTRITIONAL VALUES			
2 Carbohydrate	**Calories**	200	**Potassium**	135 mg
1 $^1/_2$ Fat	Calories from Fat	70	**Total Carbohydrate**	30 g
	Total Fat	8.0 g	Dietary Fiber	3 g
	Saturated Fat	0.8 g	Sugars	14 g
	Trans Fat	0.0 g	**Protein**	5 g
	Cholesterol	25 mg	**Phosphorus**	160 mg
	Sodium	160 mg		

Stir It Up Snacker Cake

1 (16-ounce) package sugar-free yellow
   cake mix
8 ounces club soda
$\frac{3}{4}$ **cup** egg substitute
$\frac{1}{2}$ **teaspoon** almond extract
Cooking spray
1 (15-ounce) can sliced peaches in
   100% juice, well drained and diced
2 (8-ounce cans) pineapple tidbits,
   well drained
$\frac{1}{3}$ **cup** flaked sweetened coconut or
   1$\frac{1}{2}$ **ounces** sliced almonds

1 Preheat oven to 325°F. Whisk together the cake mix,
   soda, eggs, and extract in a large bowl. Note: Batter
   will be slightly lumpy. Place in a 13 × 9-inch baking
   pan coated with cooking spray and top with peaches,
   pineapple, and coconut.

2 Bake for 45 minutes or until wooden pick inserted comes
   out clean. Cool completely on wire rack.

EXCHANGES / CHOICES
1 $\frac{1}{2}$ Carbohydrate
$\frac{1}{2}$ Fat

BASIC NUTRITIONAL VALUES

Calories	130	**Potassium**	90 mg
Calories from Fat	30	**Total Carbohydrate**	24 g
Total Fat	3.5 g	Dietary Fiber	1 g
Saturated Fat	1.7 g	Sugars	6 g
Trans Fat	0.0 g	**Protein**	3 g
Cholesterol	0 mg	**Phosphorus**	105 mg
Sodium	260 mg		

Frozen Mango Yogurt Pops

4 ounces frozen chopped mango, partially thawed

½ cup plain low-fat Greek yogurt

3 tablespoons orange juice or apricot nectar

2 tablespoons apricot or peach fruit spread

½ teaspoon vanilla extract

1 Combine all the ingredients in a blender. Puree until smooth. Pour into 4 pop molds.

2 Freeze overnight or at least 6 hours.

EXCHANGES / CHOICES

1 Fruit

BASIC NUTRITIONAL VALUES

Calories	70	**Potassium**	120 mg
Calories from Fat	10	**Total Carbohydrate**	12 g
Total Fat	1.0 g	Dietary Fiber	1 g
Saturated Fat	0.5 g	Sugars	11 g
Trans Fat	0.0 g	**Protein**	3 g
Cholesterol	0 mg	**Phosphorus**	45 mg
Sodium	15 mg		

Peanutty Pumpkin Pudding

1   Combine all ingredients, except $^1/_3$ cup of the whipped topping, in a blender and puree until smooth. Pour into 6 ramekins.

2   Refrigerate until firm according to package directions. Serve topped with the remaining whipped topping.

$^1/_2$ of a 15-ounce can solid pumpkin

1 ounce package sugar-free vanilla instant pudding and pie filling

2 cups fat-free half and half

$^1/_3$ **cup** reduced-fat creamy peanut butter

1 teaspoon vanilla extract

2 cups fat-free whipped topping

EXCHANGES / CHOICES

2 Carbohydrate
1 Fat

BASIC NUTRITIONAL VALUES

Calories	200	**Potassium**	365 mg
Calories from Fat	55	**Total Carbohydrate**	29 g
Total Fat	6.0 g	Dietary Fiber	2 g
Saturated Fat	1.4 g	Sugars	10 g
Trans Fat	0.0 g	**Protein**	5 g
Cholesterol	5 mg	**Phosphorus**	325 mg
Sodium	380 mg		

Peanut Butter Mocha Bowls

1/3 **cup** granulated sugar
3 **tablespoons** cocoa powder
2 **tablespoons** cornstarch
1 1/2 **tablespoons** instant coffee granules
2 **cups** fat-free half and half
1/4 **cup** creamy reduced-fat peanut
   butter
1/2 **teaspoon** vanilla extract
1/4 **cup plus** 2 **tablespoons** fat-free
   whipped topping

1   Whisk together the sugar, cocoa powder, cornstarch, and coffee granules in a medium saucepan. Whisk in the half and half. Bring to a boil over medium-high heat. Cook 1 minute, stirring frequently. Remove from heat.

2   Whisk in the peanut butter and vanilla, stirring until smooth. Spoon about 1/3 cup pudding into each of 6 bowls. Top each serving with whipped topping and sprinkle additional coffee granules on top.

EXCHANGES / CHOICES

2 Carbohydrate
1 Fat

BASIC NUTRITIONAL VALUES

Calories	175	**Potassium**	295 mg
Calories from Fat	45	**Total Carbohydrate**	29 g
Total Fat	5.0 g	Dietary Fiber	2 g
Saturated Fat	1.4 g	Sugars	17 g
Trans Fat	0.0 g	**Protein**	5 g
Cholesterol	5 mg	**Phosphorus**	185 mg
Sodium	150 mg		

Frozen Banana Grahams

Serves: 4
Serving Size: 1 sandwich

1 tablespoon plus 1 teaspoon creamy reduced-fat peanut butter
8 graham cracker squares (2$^{1}/_{2}$-inch squares each)
1 medium banana, cut into 16 slices
$^{1}/_{2}$ cup frozen low-fat vanilla yogurt

1 Spread the peanut butter evenly over 4 crackers (1 teaspoon each), top each with 4 banana slices, and 2 tablespoons frozen yogurt. Top with the remaining 4 crackers and press down gently to adhere.

2 Wrap each sandwich in foil and freeze overnight or at least 4 hours until firm.

Cook's Tip: May double or triple easily, but work in small batches because the yogurt melts quickly.

EXCHANGES / CHOICES

2 Carbohydrate
$^{1}/_{2}$ Fat

BASIC NUTRITIONAL VALUES

Calories	145	**Potassium**	205 mg
Calories from Fat	35	**Total Carbohydrate**	25 g
Total Fat	4.0 g	Dietary Fiber	2 g
Saturated Fat	1.0 g	Sugars	12 g
Trans Fat	0.0 g	**Protein**	3 g
Cholesterol	0 mg	**Phosphorus**	65 mg
Sodium	130 mg		

Berry, Walnut, and Oat Crumble

SERVES: 8
SERVING SIZE: 1/2 cup crumble mixture and 2 tablespoons yogurt

1 1/2 tablespoons lemon juice
1 tablespoon vanilla
2 tablespoon cornstarch
4 cups fresh or frozen, thawed mixed berries

Topping

2/3 cup quick-cooking oats
2 ounces chopped walnuts
1/2 cup sugar
2 tablespoons canola oil
1/2 teaspoon ground cinnamon
1/8 teaspoon salt
1 cup nonfat plain Greek yogurt (optional)

1 Preheat oven to 350°F. Meanwhile, in a 2-quart casserole dish, stir together lemon juice, vanilla, and cornstarch until cornstarch is dissolved. Stir in the berries.

2 Stir together the topping ingredients in a medium bowl until crumbled texture. Sprinkle evenly over the berries and bake, uncovered, for 30 minutes.

COOK'S TIP: For a browner topping, remove the crumble, heat the broiler, and run under broiler 1–2 minutes, being careful not to burn.

EXCHANGES / CHOICES	BASIC NUTRITIONAL VALUES			
2 Carbohydrate	**Calories**	195	**Potassium**	160 mg
1 1/2 Fat	Calories from Fat	80	**Total Carbohydrate**	28 g
	Total Fat	9.0 g	Dietary Fiber	4 g
	Saturated Fat	0.8 g	Sugars	18 g
	Trans Fat	0.0 g	**Protein**	3 g
	Cholesterol	0 mg	**Phosphorus**	70 mg
	Sodium	40 mg		

SERVES: 8
SERVING SIZE: 1 slice

4 cups frozen low-fat vanilla yogurt
16 chocolate wafers, crushed
1 tablespoon instant coffee granules
16 sugar-free peppermints, crushed

1 Spoon the yogurt into a 9-inch pie pan. (May want to use a fork to spread evenly.) Sprinkle the crushed cookies evenly over all and sprinkle with the coffee granules and the peppermints.

2 Cover and freeze overnight.

COOK'S TIP: Frozen yogurt thaws faster than traditional ice cream; let stand 5 minutes on kitchen counter before slicing.

EXCHANGES / CHOICES	BASIC NUTRITIONAL VALUES			
2 Carbohydrate	**Calories**	180	**Potassium**	170 mg
½ Fat	Calories from Fat	25	**Total Carbohydrate**	34 g
	Total Fat	3.0 g	Dietary Fiber	1 g
	Saturated Fat	2.0 g	Sugars	18 g
	Trans Fat	0.0 g	**Protein**	4 g
	Cholesterol	10 mg	**Phosphorus**	110 mg
	Sodium	110 mg		

Layered Strawberry-Banana Pudding

2 **cups** fat-free milk

1 (1-ounce) package vanilla sugar-free, fat-free instant pudding mix

2 **cups** fat-free whipped topping

¹/₂ **cup** nonfat plain Greek yogurt

2 **teaspoons** vanilla extract

20 reduced-fat vanilla wafers

1 ripe medium banana, thinly sliced

1 ¹/₂ **cups** sliced strawberries

1 Whisk together the milk and pudding mix in a large bowl until well blended. Whisk in the whipped topping, yogurt, and vanilla until smooth.

2 Arrange the cookies in a single layer in the bottom of an 11 × 7-inch baking pan. Spoon half of the pudding mixture evenly over the cookies, top with the bananas, remaining pudding mixture, and sprinkle the strawberries evenly over all. Cover and refrigerate overnight or at least 8 hours.

COOK'S TIP: If an 11 × 7-inch baking dish is not available, you may use a shallow 2-quart casserole dish, and overlap the cookies slightly.

EXCHANGES / CHOICES	BASIC NUTRITIONAL VALUES			
2 Carbohydrate	**Calories**	140	**Potassium**	250 mg
	Calories from Fat	10	**Total Carbohydrate**	27 g
	Total Fat	1.0 g	Dietary Fiber	1 g
	Saturated Fat	0.1 g	Sugars	14 g
	Trans Fat	0.0 g	**Protein**	4 g
	Cholesterol	0 mg	**Phosphorus**	205 mg
	Sodium	230 mg		

Cinnamon Raspberry Cookie Cake Squares

SERVES: 24
SERVING SIZE: 1 (2-inch) square

1 Preheat oven to 350°F. Meanwhile, stir together the cake mix, eggs, and all but 2 tablespoons of the oil in a large bowl. Spread mixture evenly over the bottom of a 13 × 9-inch nonstick baking pan coated with cooking spray. (Note: For easier spreading, coat a rubber spatula or the back of a large spoon with cooking spray.) Top evenly with the frozen berries.

2 In the same bowl used to combine the cake mix, stir together the oats, the remaining 2 tablespoons oil, almonds, sugar, and cinnamon to a crumble texture. Sprinkle evenly over the cake and bake 25 minutes or until wooden pick inserted comes out clean. Cool completely on wire rack, before cutting into squares.

1 (16-ounce) box sugar-free yellow cake mix
³/₄ **cup** egg substitute
¹/₂ **cup** canola oil, divided use
4 cups frozen raspberries
¹/₂ **cup** quick-cooking oats
3 ounces slivered almonds, coarsely crumbled
¹/₄ **cup** sugar
2 teaspoons ground cinnamon

COOK'S TIP: The texture and flavors are even better next day.

EXCHANGES / CHOICES
1 Carbohydrate
1¹/₂ Fat

BASIC NUTRITIONAL VALUES

Calories	155	**Potassium**	105 mg
Calories from Fat	70	**Total Carbohydrate**	19 g
Total Fat	8.0 g	Dietary Fiber	1 g
Saturated Fat	1.1 g	Sugars	6 g
Trans Fat	0.0 g	**Protein**	3 g
Cholesterol	0 mg	**Phosphorus**	95 mg
Sodium	160 mg		

Sangria Shaved Ice

SERVES: 15
SERVING SIZE: $^2/_3$ cup

3 cups dry red wine
3 cups orange juice
1 (12-ounce) can or **1 $^1/_2$ cups** diet ginger ale
$^1/_2$ cup sugar
2 tablespoons lemon juice
2 tablespoons lime juice

1   Combine all the ingredients in a gallon-size resealable plastic bag or other airtight container. Seal tightly and shake gently back and forth until well blended. Freeze overnight. (Note: if using a resealable bag, place on a baking sheet on its side for support.)

2   When frozen, shave with fork or break up large pieces with a knife, reseal the baggie, and crush with your hands to create a "slush" effect. Store unused portion in freezer.

COOK'S TIP: May replace wine with 3 cups cranberry juice and use $^1/_3$ cup sugar. If using juice, the frozen mixture will have to stand on kitchen counter 20 minutes to soften slightly and be shaved each time. The wine mixture will remain a "shaved" texture when returned to the freezer because of the alcohol.

EXCHANGES / CHOICES
1 Carbohydrate

BASIC NUTRITIONAL VALUES

Calories	85	**Potassium**	155 mg
Calories from Fat	0	**Total Carbohydrate**	13 g
Total Fat	0.0 g	Dietary Fiber	0 g
Saturated Fat	0.0 g	Sugars	12 g
Trans Fat	0.0 g	**Protein**	0 g
Cholesterol	0 mg	**Phosphorus**	15 mg
Sodium	5 mg		

Sweet Blueberry Lime Crème Pots

SERVES: 6
SERVING SIZE: $1/3$ cup cream mixture, 2 tablespoons crumbs, and $1/4$ cup berries

1 Whisk together the yogurt, cream cheese, sugar, lime zest, juice, and vanilla in a medium bowl until smooth. Gently stir in the whipped topping until just blended.

2 Place equal amounts of the berries in the bottom of 6 ramekins and spoon the lime mixture on top. Cover with plastic wrap and refrigerate overnight or at least 8 hours. Serve topped with the cracker crumbs.

1 (5.3-ounce) container nonfat vanilla Greek yogurt
1 ounce whipped cream cheese spread, softened*
3 tablespoons sugar
$1/2$ teaspoon grated lime zest
2 tablespoons lime juice
1 teaspoon vanilla extract
$1^1/2$ cups fat-free whipped topping
$1^1/2$ cups fresh or frozen, thawed blueberries
6 (2 × 2-inch squared) low-fat graham crackers, coarsely crumbled

*COOK'S TIP: To soften quickly, place the cream cheese on a microwave-safe plate and microwave on high setting for 20 seconds.

EXCHANGES / CHOICES
2 Carbohydrate

BASIC NUTRITIONAL VALUES

Calories	140	Potassium	90 mg
Calories from Fat	20	Total Carbohydrate	27 g
Total Fat	2.0 g	Dietary Fiber	1 g
Saturated Fat	0.7 g	Sugars	15 g
Trans Fat	0.0 g	Protein	3 g
Cholesterol	5 mg	Phosphorus	60 mg
Sodium	90 mg		

DESSERTS

Peaches on Whipped Raspberry Cream

SERVES: 4
SERVING SIZE: $1/4$ cup raspberry cream mixture and $1/2$ cup sliced peaches

4 ounces fat-free cream cheese, softened*
$1/4$ cup raspberry fruit spread
1 tablespoon lower-fat (<50% vegetable oil) margarine-type spread
1 tablespoon lime juice
1 teaspoon granulated sugar
$1/2$ teaspoon vanilla extract
$1/4$ teaspoon almond extract
$1/2$ cup fat-free whipped topping
2 cups sliced peaches or nectarines

1 Whisk together the cream cheese, fruit spread, margarine, lime juice, sugar, and extracts in a medium bowl until smooth. Gently stir in the whipped topping until just blended. Spoon into 4 dessert bowls, cover, and refrigerate overnight or at least 4 hours.

2 Spoon equal amounts of the peaches over each serving of raspberry cream.

*COOK'S TIP: To soften quickly, place the cream cheese on a microwave-safe plate and microwave on high setting for 20 seconds.

EXCHANGES / CHOICES	BASIC NUTRITIONAL VALUES			
$1 1/2$ Carbohydrate	**Calories**	130	**Potassium**	255 mg
$1/2$ Fat	Calories from Fat	15	**Total Carbohydrate**	23 g
	Total Fat	1.5 g	Dietary Fiber	1 g
	Saturated Fat	0.3 g	Sugars	18 g
	Trans Fat	0.0 g	**Protein**	4 g
	Cholesterol	5 mg	**Phosphorus**	175 mg
	Sodium	215 mg		

Pink Peppermint Strawberry Sauce

1 Combine the strawberries, candies, water, and extract in a medium bowl.

2 Cover and refrigerate 1 hour. (Note: the mixture will thicken slightly.) May serve over frozen low-fat vanilla yogurt or ripe pear slices or angel food cake.

Sauce

2 cups diced strawberries

24 sugar-free peppermint hard candies, crushed in baggie

1/4 cup water

1/4 teaspoon peppermint extract

EXCHANGES / CHOICES

1 Carbohydrate

BASIC NUTRITIONAL VALUES

Calories	45	**Potassium**	65 mg
Calories from Fat	0	**Total Carbohydrate**	11 g
Total Fat	0.0 g	Dietary Fiber	1 g
Saturated Fat	0.0 g	Sugars	2 g
Trans Fat	0.0 g	**Protein**	0 g
Cholesterol	0 mg	**Phosphorus**	10 mg
Sodium	0 mg		

Mexican Chocolate, Zucchini, and Cinnamon Squares

SERVES: 18
SERVING SIZE: 3 × 2-inch piece

1 (16-ounce) package sugar-free devil's
   food cake mix
3/4 **cup** egg substitute
2 medium zucchini, shredded
1/2 **cup** water
3 **tablespoons** canola oil
1 1/2 **tablespoons** instant coffee granules
1 teaspoon ground cinnamon
1/2 **teaspoon** almond extract
3 **ounces** chopped pecans

1 Preheat oven to 325°F. Meanwhile, combine all the ingredients in a large bowl. Using an electric mixer on medium speed, beat 2 minutes. Pour into a nonstick 13 × 9-inch cake pan coated with cooking spray and bake 28 minutes or until wooden pick inserted comes out almost clean.

2 Remove from oven, place pan on cooling rack, and cool completely.

COOK'S TIP: This is one of those recipes that just gets more moist as the days go by . . . may store at room temperature up to 3 days or freeze a portion for a later use.

COOK'S TIP: Use a food processor to shred zucchini superfast!

EXCHANGES / CHOICES	BASIC NUTRITIONAL VALUES			
1 1/2 Carbohydrate	Calories	145	Potassium	180 mg
1 Fat	Calories from Fat	70	**Total Carbohydrate**	21 g
	Total Fat	8.0 g	Dietary Fiber	2 g
	Saturated Fat	1.5 g	Sugars	1 g
	Trans Fat	0.0 g	**Protein**	3 g
	Cholesterol	0 mg	**Phosphorus**	95 mg
	Sodium	195 mg		

INDEX

Alphabetical Index

Subject Index

Metric Equivalents

Liquid Measurement	Metric equivalent
1 teaspoon	5 mL
1 tablespoon *or* 1/2 fluid ounce	15 mL
1 fluid ounce *or* 1/8 cup	30 mL
1/4 cup *or* 2 fluid ounces	60 mL
1/3 cup	80 mL
1/2 cup *or* 4 fluid ounces	120 mL
2/3 cup	160 mL
3/4 cup *or* 6 fluid ounces	180 mL
1 cup *or* 8 fluid ounces *or* 1/2 pint	240 mL
1 1/2 cups *or* 12 fluid ounces	350 mL
2 cups *or* 1 pint *or* 16 fluid ounces	475 mL
3 cups *or* 1 1/2 pints	700 mL
4 cups *or* 2 pints *or* 1 quart	950 mL
4 quarts *or* 1 gallon	3.8 L

Weight Measurement	Metric equivalent
1 ounce	28 g
4 ounces *or* 1/4 pound	113 g
1/3 pound	150 g
8 ounces *or* 1/2 pound	230 g
2/3 pound	300 g
12 ounces *or* 3/4 pound	340 g
1 pound *or* 16 ounces	450 g
2 pounds	900 g

Dry Measurements	Metric equivalent
1 teaspoon	5 g
1 tablespoon	14 g
1/4 cup	57 g
1/2 cup	113 g
3/4 cup	168 g
1 cup	224 g

Length	Metric equivalent
1/8 inch	3 mm
1/4 inch	6 mm
1/2 inch	13 mm
3/4 inch	19 mm
1 inch	2.5 cm
2 inches	5 cm

Fahrenheit	Celsius
275°F	140°C
300°F	150°C
325°F	165°C
350°F	180°C
375°F	190°C

Fahrenheit	Celsius
400°F	200°C
425°F	220°C
450°F	230°C
475°F	240°C
500°F	260°C

Weights of common ingredients in grams							
Ingredient	1 cup	3/4 cup	2/3 cup	1/2 cup	1/3 cup	1/4 cup	2 Tbsp
Flour, all-purpose (wheat)	120 g	90 g	80 g	60 g	40 g	30 g	15 g
Flour, well-sifted, all-purpose (wheat)	110 g	80 g	70 g	55 g	35 g	27 g	13 g
Sugar, granulated cane	200 g	150 g	130 g	100 g	65 g	50 g	25 g
Confectioner's sugar (cane)	100 g	75 g	70 g	50 g	35 g	25 g	13 g
Brown sugar, packed firmly	180 g	135 g	120 g	90 g	60 g	45 g	23 g
Cornmeal	160 g	120 g	100 g	80 g	50 g	40 g	20 g
Cornstarch	120 g	90 g	80 g	60 g	40 g	30 g	15 g
Rice, uncooked	190 g	140 g	125 g	95 g	65 g	48 g	24 g
Macaroni, uncooked	140 g	100 g	90 g	70 g	45 g	35 g	17 g
Couscous, uncooked	180 g	135 g	120 g	90 g	60 g	45 g	22 g
Oats, uncooked, quick	90 g	65 g	60 g	45 g	30 g	22 g	11 g
Table salt	300 g	230 g	200 g	150 g	100 g	75 g	40 g
Butter	240 g	180 g	160 g	120 g	80 g	60 g	30 g
Vegetable shortening	190 g	140 g	125 g	95 g	65 g	48 g	24 g
Chopped fruits and vegetables	150 g	110 g	100 g	75 g	50 g	40 g	20 g
Nuts, chopped	150 g	110 g	100 g	75 g	50 g	40 g	20 g
Nuts, ground	120 g	90 g	80 g	60 g	40 g	30 g	15 g
Bread crumbs, fresh, loosely packed	60 g	45 g	40 g	30 g	20 g	15 g	8 g
Bread crumbs, dry	150 g	110 g	100 g	75 g	50 g	40 g	20 g
Parmesan cheese, grated	90 g	65 g	60 g	45 g	30 g	22 g	11 g